INTERPRETING AND HOLDING

INTERPRETING AND HOLDING

The Paternal and Maternal Functions of the Psychotherapist

JEFFREY SEINFELD, PH.D.

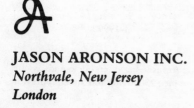

JASON ARONSON INC.
Northvale, New Jersey
London

Production Editor: Judith D. Cohen

This book was set in 11 pt. Bem by Lind Graphics of Upper Saddle River, New Jersey, and printed and bound by Haddon Craftsmen of Scranton, Pennsylvania.

Copyright © 1993 by Jason Aronson Inc.

10 9 8 7 6 5 4 3 2 1

Library of Congress Cataloging-in-Publication Data

Seinfeld, Jeffrey.
    Interpreting and holding : the paternal and maternal functions
of the psychotherapist / by Jeffrey Seinfeld.
      p. cm.
    Includes bibliographical references and index.
    ISBN 0-87668-501-7
    1. Psychotherapy. 2. Psychotherapist and patient.
3. Psychoanalytic interpretation. 4. Object relations
(Psychoanalysis) 5. Regression (Psychology)—Therapeutic use.
6. Mother and child. 7. Father and child. I. Title.
    [DNLM: 1. Psychoanalytic Interpretation. 2. Physician's Role.
3. Physician–Patient Relations. WM 460.7 S461i 1993]
RC480.5.S4165   1993
616.89′ 14—dc20
DNLM/DLC
for Library of Congress   93-19992

Manufactured in the United States of America. Jason Aronson Inc. offers books and cassettes. For information and catalog write to Jason Aronson Inc., 230 Livingston Street, Northvale, New Jersey 07647.

To
Albert, Frieda, Barbara, and Michael

Contents

Acknowledgment

I would like to express my appreciation to my wife Rhonda and my daughter Leonora for their support and encouragement.

I would like to thank Jason Aronson, M.D., and his editorial staff for their support and encouragement. Dean Shirley Ehrenkranz, Dr. George Frank, Dr. Burt Shachter, Dr. Eda Goldstein, Dr. Gladys Gonzales-Ramos, Dr. Judith Siegel, Dr. Theresa Aiello-Gerber and the entire NYU faculty were important sources of collegiality, encouragement, and support. My thanks goes to Mrs. Pat Nitzburg, Mrs. Rita Smith, and the participants in the ongoing clinical workshops of the Jewish Board of Family and Children's Services for their strong support. I am especially grateful to Mr. Robert Berger for his unwavering support. I am grateful to Dr. Michael Gropper, Ms. Charna Meyers, Ms. Cheri Lieberman, and Ms. Diane Cullen for their support and encouragement. I am grateful to Mr. Mordecai Mandelbaum for his excellent clinical material and thoughtful ideas.

PART ONE

INTERPRETING

1

FREUD AND THE PATERNAL MODE OF THERAPY

THE POSITION OF THE FATHER

Sigmund Freud and D. W. Winnicott exemplify the paternal and maternal functions of the psychotherapist, respectively. Both parental modes are necessary to therapy, and both contribute to the creation of the symbolic forms of the self. Hegel taught that it is impossible to understand one aspect of a dialectic without comparison with its counterpart. Therefore, although this chapter is about Freud and the paternal mode of therapy, I will have occasion to speak of the maternal function, which will be fully discussed in its own right later.

Freud's metaphor for analysis is that of a chess game or of war with strategies to overcome the patient's resistances and defenses. Kenneth Wright (1991c) points out that Freud's personality and position are predominantly paternal in that the struggle with his father is at the center of this personality and his therapeutic stance. Freud identifies with the position of the father as stern, forbidding, and prohibiting, the guardian of the reality principle. Ernest Jones states that Freud identified with Moses, the father of the Jewish people, the Deliverer and the Guardian of the Law. There is an emphasis on therapy as work, a battle to be fought against resistances, a triumph to be won.

5

In *Remembering, Repeating and Working Through* (1914), Freud discusses the struggle with the patient "to keep in the psychical sphere all the impulses which his patient would like to direct into the motor sphere" (p. 373). The goal of analysis is for the patient to remember and to put all impulses into words. However, the patient is incapable of remembering and instead repeats. Repetition tends toward action, not awareness or verbalization. What the patient cannot remember are thoughts that merely have the possibility of existing but have never been symbolized. Instead they are expressed in feelings, expectations, and behavior.

Wright (1992d) points out that the therapist must enable the patient to stand off from what he feels or has an impulse to do, to hold it in the mind, rather than enact it, reject it, or discharge it. Freud struggled to preserve a space of separateness for the patient to explore and understand his patterns of feelings, relationships, and experience. Wright compares the patient's holding off from action to the child's separation from the caregiving object, both of which are an essential precondition to symbol formation. A space is thereby created where an object can be conceived, held, and contemplated without seeking direct satisfaction from it. Wright (1991d) says,

> From this point of view, the analytic space can be thought of as a space in which symbols are (to be) formed; the "no action" rule, which the analyst, where necessary, struggles to preserve, is protective of this function. It is not, however, a space for forming symbols in general, but a space for forming symbols of the self. *It is a space in which a self that was blindly lived will be transformed, through the analytic looking, into a self that is conceivable, a self that is known.* [p. 286]

In observing transference love, Freud described a situation in which both the analytic and psychic space are not holding. The therapist struggles "to keep in the psychical sphere all the impulses which his patient would like to direct in the motor sphere." This gives way to a rejection of symbolization. The need for direct satisfaction with the object has proved overwhelming. The mind, lacking a recollected maternal presence, becomes an empty core. Its need is therefore to be filled with concrete internal objects because it cannot tolerate symbolic objects. Freud responded to this situation by reinforcing the failing boundary with paternal prohibition and interpretations. Wright (1991d) states, "The object must be given up. It is the oedipal imperative, which guarantees a space for the world" (p. 285).

Wright says that the position of the father, the third position, is important in considering symbol formation and therapy. Once the earlier maternal space of symbolic formation, that of playing with patterns of objects, is well established, the third position of the father allows for a greater expansion of vision, enhancing the range and variety of patterns that can be seen and used and letting the child explore the large world opened up by the father.

In the beginning of therapy, the therapist is experienced as someone outside the patient's life. He occupies the third position, an observer of the patient's life, a position held by the father in relation to the mother–infant pair. However, it is not long before the therapist becomes an attachment figure who is part of the patient's life and no longer an outside observer of it. This promises a recreation of the original dyadic situation. The patient is here longing for a love object to put right the wrongs of the past. The patient seeks direct gratification and fears rejection. By virtue of the therapist's caring and supportive attitude, he or she becomes the object of unfulfilled longings and disappointments that have shaped the patient. Wright (1991d) states, "Yet in a certain sense, the therapist's chair is always empty. At the moment when the patient would look for his longing to be satisfied, the therapist is not there; he will not provide the satisfaction" (p. 299). The therapist is a nobody, a blank screen. As the feeling of intimacy revives the patient's deepest longings for the mother, the therapist interprets the patient's wishes. He is suddenly no longer there but is instead in the third position, outside the mother–infant dyad, inviting the patient to join him there to look and understand. In the paternal function, the therapist is outside the mother–infant dyad in a place from which the dyad can be seen so that the therapist can provide insight and knowledge.

In contrast to the paternal function, Winnicott represents the therapist as mother. He replaces the metaphor of therapy as work with that of therapy as play. Ferenczi, and Alice and Michael Balint were earlier analysts in this tradition. They had the courage and conviction to stand up to the father and insist on the place of the mother. As Wright points out, Winnicott stands for loving, caring, and providing a more lenient space and protection from the impingement of reality. Freud describes a patient uninterested in insight, who tries to obliviate the therapeutic space that Freud guards. This is the space of separateness where symbols of the self are formed. Freud insists on maintaining a radical gap. Winnicott's patient, in contrast, is not bent on obliterating the space but is intent on exploring and patterning things within the holding environment of the therapist mother. Winnicott's patient at the moment is not seeking satisfaction. Instead, the patient relates in a pattern-matching way without trying to possess the therapist. Freud insists on a radical separateness and otherness, whereas Winnicott permits the patient to play in potential space.

THE CENTRALITY OF THE OEDIPAL CONFLICT AND THE FEAR OF SUCCESS

Freud based his theories primarily on the study of the development of the male child. Only after prolonged study of the centrality of the Oedipus conflict did psychoanalysis concern itself with the infant–mother dyad that is central to the formation and development of the self. In the discussion of the oedipal conflict, Freud focused on the competition and hatred that the little boy felt for the father in competing for the love of the mother. The castration complex was crucial in accounting for the resolution of the oedipal complex. It was the child's recognition of the anatomical differences between the sexes that originally brought about castration anxiety. Wright maintains that in the oedipal moment, the child feels that he has lost both parents and that they exist for each other instead of for him, or at least not only for him. The child must gradually allow for the parents to be together in this psychic space without intruding on them. The child must learn to look but not to do in relationship to the oedipal parental couple. Jacques Lacan (1955) referred to the possessive father upholding the parental boundary with the threat of castration, which he described with the metaphor "the Law of the Father." This absolute incest boundary has been noted by Levi-Strauss as the basis of culture. Wright finds that it is the achievement of the oedipal space that allows for the inner world of language, thought, and representation, the realm of the logos that is forever separated from the sensorial thing world it represents. As the oedipal couple can be seen or contemplated but not touched, the world remains ungraspable except by thought. I agree with Wright (1991c) that Lacan may have meant this in stating that "the father, or the name-of-the-father, stands at the entry to the symbolic order" (p. 126).

Freud saw the psychoneurosis as a retreat from the anxieties of the oedipal conflict to earlier pregenital levels of libidinal conflict. The patient was also viewed as resisting the analyst's efforts to create a radical space of separateness from the oedipal mother. Lacan's "Law of the Father" refers to the concept of the paternal function as separation from the oedipal mother. This idea is illustrated in the following vignette.

An adult male patient raised in the Orthodox Jewish tradition reports to me that on the way to his session he was looking at pretty women and kiddingly thinking that if he had all of them as lovers, he would not need therapy. This brought to mind a recurring fantasy of his adolescence. He imagined being in the synagogue studying the Law of God. The men and women were seated separately. Custom had it that the women wore dresses with long sleeves and high necklines. A naked, beautiful woman entered the synagogue, coming to him seductively, draping herself over him. The men he was studying with were shocked, confused, and in turmoil. After telling me this fantasy, the patient recalls a dream. There is a maid who has been with his family during his childhood and adolescence. He is in bed and she joins him naked. She gets on top and he desires her but thinks she could have AIDS. In fear, he flees.

I interpret that the Law of the Father is represented both by the therapist and by the Law of God. At first, the patient announces he wants to be with all the women he sees on the way to therapy so that he will no longer need therapy, then he defies the Law of God in fantasy by having the naked woman interrupt the study of the Law. The woman again appears as the maid, closer to being recognized as the oedipal mother because she took care of the patient in his childhood and he thought of her as a second mother. The fear of AIDS is a return of the Law of the Father, symbolizing castration and prohibiting and preventing incest.

Freud (1915) believed that for a neurosis to occur, there must be a conflict between the libidinal desires of the person and that part of his being that expresses the interests of reality and morality. A pathogenic conflict typically occurs when the libido wishes to pursue gratification unacceptable to the ego but instead encounters frustration and privation. Freud remarked on those surprising cases that fell ill, not out of frustration but rather because a deeply rooted, long-cherished wish comes to fulfillment. He felt that such patients are wrecked by success and cannot endure their bliss. Freud elaborated that in those cases where frustration gives rise to neurosis, it is not actually pathogenic until there is an internal frustration as well. In other words, the ego joins hands with the external frustration and disputes the rights of the libido toward other objects it also wishes to possess. It is at this point that substitute gratification proceeds by way of the unconscious circuitously giving rise to neurotic symptoms. In cases where neurotic symptoms follow success, only the internal frustration operates. It makes its appearance not as a result of an external frustration but rather following the fulfillment of a wish. Freud explained this seemingly astounding phenomenon by pointing out that the ego tolerates a wish as harmless far more readily as long as it exists in fantasy with little or no opportunity for gratification. The wish becomes a much greater threat when external circumstances permit its opportunity for fulfillment.

Freud (1915) described a professor at a university who for many years longed to succeed the master who had initiated him into the life of learning. When the elder man retired and the younger man's colleagues suggested that he was next in line as successor, he hesitated, depreciated his own merits, said he was unworthy, and fell into a state of depression that left him debilitated.

The patient's success neurosis could be understood in this way: succeeding the master represented killing the father and winning the mother (the longed-for position). Thus, success was forbidden because it unconsciously signified defying the Law of the Father.

A female adult patient I treated had a lifelong school and work inhibition but secretly dreamed of being a writer. She eventually took courses at the university and received an A for a paper she had written. She was fearful of the envious reaction of the other students but attempted to cover over this conflict by constantly putting herself in a position of allowing them to take advantage of her. As long as she served them, she could avoid their envy. Receiving an excellent grade from the teacher signified being loved by the father, for which the oedipal mother would retaliate.

THE INTERPRETIVE TECHNIQUE

Psychoanalytic technique evolved from the method of abreaction, whereby the therapist directed the patient's attention to the events that gave rise to symptom formation, to the receding of abreaction and the concentration of treatment on the patient's conscious resistances so that he could pursue free associations. Freud (1914) came upon the classical technique whereby the analyst permitted the patient to freely follow any and all trains of thought and utilized interpretation to recognize and overcome resistances. Freud's interpretive technique increasingly focused on the patient's tendency to repeat and enact, as opposed to remember, what is forgotten and repressed. It is here that Freud developed the dictum that the patient must put all inner thoughts, feelings, fantasies, and impulses into words and not actions.

Freud became aware that the patient did not recall or describe how defiant he was of his parents' authority but instead behaved that way toward the analyst. He did not recall his shame over sexual matters, but was ashamed of the treatment and kept it a secret. Freud (1914) recommended that the analyst begin treatment by announcing the fundamental rule and that the patient say whatever comes to mind, however seemingly irrelevant, shameful, or trivial. The patient typically responds by having nothing to say. However,

the patient cannot escape "the compulsion to repeat" (p. 370).
Freud emphasized that the compulsion to repeat was the transference of the repressed past not only onto the analyst but onto every
aspect of the current situation. Resistance was thus comprised by
the substitution of action for recollection.

Freud recommended that the analyst encourage the patient to
pay attention to all details of his symptoms and problems: What are
the exact words and impulses of his obsessive ideas? Under what
situations does his phobia occur? The patient is supported in becoming tolerant of his condition. Freud pointed out that the patient's increased tolerance could result in an exacerbation of
symptoms. He advised the therapist to assure the patient that this is
only a temporary and necessary outbreak that allows for the
symptom or "enemy" to be in range and thereby be overcome.
Freud (1914) stated that the therapist is in a "perpetual struggle
with the patient to keep all the impulses which he would like to
carry into action within the boundaries of his mind, and when it is
possible to divert into the work of recollection any impulse which
the patient wants to discharge in action" (p. 373). He recommended
making the patient promise not to carry out any important life
decisions during the treatment concerning choice of a permanent
love object or profession, but to postpone such decisions until after
termination. He feared that the patient might act out, instead of
recall, repressed memories. However, he also recognized that there
was often nothing to do but allow certain patients to act out because
only afterwards would they be willing to analyze the impulse or
action.

In fact, Freud cautioned therapists from interpreting the resistance prematurely. The patient must be allowed time to get to
know, experience, and recognize the resistance. He recommended
interpreting the resistance only after it has run its course and is at its
height. In fact, Freud took an increasingly cautious attitude in
respect to the timing of interpretations. He said that the transference
should be left untouched until the transference resistance appeared
and that the analyst should not attempt to disclose to patients the
hidden meaning of their thoughts or feelings until a dependable,
positive transference or rapport is established. He revealed that in

earlier years, he learned that premature interpretation often brought the treatment to a premature termination.

Freud (1905) found that the patient himself revealed the appropriate time for interpretation when he suffered under an exaggerated or pressured train of thought. The intensity of the patient's feelings suggested that they were reinforced by unconscious concerns, and the therapist could then interest the patient in exploring the unconscious.

The classical technique was aimed at uncovering oedipal conflict, often a psychosexual retreat from the fear of oedipal success and ensuing guilt and fear of punishment. Although Freud's primary technique was interpretive, he endeavored to provide support through the timing of interventions and the education of the patient on the process of treatment.

THE INTERNALIZATION OF THE OBJECT AND DEPRESSIVE STATES

Freud discovered the resolution of the oedipal conflict in terms he first put forward in *Mourning and Melancholia* (1917). He stated there that the ego reacts to the loss of the love object by giving up the libidinal love for the object. The ego then incorporates and identifies with the lost love object. Freud's patient, the Wolfman, once remarked that Freud was an avid reader of Sherlock Holmes stories because the master sleuth's method of deduction resembled the master analyst's method of uncovering. Freud was intrigued by the mystery of why the depressive patient would be eager to tell anyone willing to listen what a despicable or loathsome person he or she was. It seemed to Freud that the depressive would be more likely to hide in shame and not want anyone to know how unworthy he was. It was this clue that led Freud to the discovery that the depressive actually ridiculed the lost object in ridiculing himself; he had incorporated and identified with the lost love object, and therefore when he shouted from the rooftops how unworthy he was the depressive was in actuality informing on the object, not himself. Freud (1917) introduced the line of thought referred to today as object relations theory in the remark "the shadow of the object fell upon the ego" (p. 159).

I will illustrate this dynamic of the depressive with a brief vignette.

A female adult patient was regularly late for her therapy sessions. It was also typical that she reproached herself for her lack of responsibility and inconsideration for coming late. The self-reproaches seemed as much a symptom as the lateness since it had no effect on changing her behavior. On one occasion, the patient talked about her childhood and happened to mention that her mother regularly brought her late for school, medical appointments, and play dates. I asked how she had felt about that and she said relieved; these activities had all created anxiety, and therefore she had been in no hurry to get to them. I pointed out that her current pattern told a different tale. She brought herself late, as her mother had taken her everywhere late, and she now said about herself-mother that she was irresponsible, lazy, and inconsiderate. The patient's mother had died several years ago and she had never mourned. In fact, she was still relating completely within the dyad of infant–mother though the object was internal. I therefore interpreted from the position of the third, inviting the patient to come out of the dyad to have a look from my standpoint.

In describing the resolution of the oedipal conflict, Freud (1917) used the same explanation he had provided for depression in *Mourning and Melancholia*. There is an identification with a lost parental object. The object is incorporated and becomes a precipitate of the ego, standing over and above it and thereby termed the superego. Freud drew upon his theory of the negative oedipal conflict to explain that the rival parent is also a libidinal love object and therefore internalized as such. Nevertheless, Freud emphasized that it is the fear of castration that motivates the child to renounce his oedipal longings. Fairbairn, Jacobson, and Wright have suggested that it is not only out of fear but also out of love for the rival parent that the patient renounces oedipal longings. Wright maintains that the renunciation of the oedipal conflict allows for the patterning of the relationship with both parents in reality, that grants to the parents their own space that excludes the child.

THE ROLE OF THE FATHER

Wright (1991c) states that the positive value that the preoedipal father serves for both sexes is not given enough attention in the psychoanalytic literature. The father exerts a positive attraction for the child in drawing him out of the symbiotic relationship with the mother. In speaking of the absence of the father, Wright means more than the physical aspect. A father may be striving to be more of a mother to the child, competing with the actual mother and thereby depriving the child of the experience of difference, or the father may be too weak or uninvolved to help the child to separate. There may have been too early a disruption of maternal symbiosis, forcing the child to turn to the father as a substitute mother to try to recreate the lost symbiosis.

For the baby in the beginning there is only the mother. The father plays a supportive rule, but the baby is unaware of him in the background. When the father serves as a substitute mother, he remains a mother or primary caregiver and does not yet fulfill a function in his own right. It is when separation occurs between the baby and the mother that the infant discovers the father as other, outside the symbiotic orbit. The father is outside the infant–mother couple in the position of the observer. The infant discovers the father as the third party in the outside observing position and experiences him both as a force drawing the infant out of the symbiosis and as an intrusion.

Wright illustrates this change in the infant's point of view by comparing it with astronauts' experience leaving the earth. He draws on Kevin Kelley's summary of the effect on astronauts of seeing the earth from outer space. In *The Home Planet—Images and Reflections of Earth from Space Explorers* (1988) Kelley found that the astronauts saw the planet with new eyes. This resulted in powerful, life-transforming changes. The astronauts had a new perception of the earth as a whole, small, bounded, fragile planet located in a much larger context. It no longer seemed limitless, vast, and invulnerable. Wright suggests that by substituting mother for the planet Earth and father for the position in space from which a new view can be obtained, we get some idea of the transforming and transformative experience of the child as it is first able to move in

imagination to the position of the third person in a triangular
relationship and to look at his earlier lived relationship from the
outside position. The child living in the dyadic relationship is
immersed in its immediacy, the mother being the limit and horizon
of its experience, limitless and invulnerable, the provider or
thwarter of satisfaction. The child can now look at itself and the
mother and see a new type of unit, one object within a larger
context of objects. In discussing the formation of groups, Jean-Paul
Sartre, in *The Critique of Dialectical Reason* (1960), writes, "The unity
of a dyad can be realized only within a totalization performed from
outside by a third party" (p. 115). Wright draws on Sartre's phenomenology to describe how the infant comes to identify with the
father in seeing itself and the mother from a third mediating position.

Mahler and colleagues (1975) suggest that with the child's
beginning capacity for motility, the father serves an important role
in helping the child to differentiate from a state of oneness with the
mother. Wright emphasizes that the father is differentiated from
the mother prior to the oedipal phase. He maintains that it is the
difference of the father from the mother that is central to the paternal
function that aids separation. He states,

> [The father] will be loved and hated for the different things he
> provides, the different way he does things. He picks me up
> differently; he swings me around; he is more exciting. He is
> someone who is not always there like mother, but who comes and
> goes; when he comes and plays with me, perhaps in a different
> way from mother, he feels different, his voice is different, he tells
> me off more sharply, and so on. The details do not matter, it is the
> *difference* that does. [p. 13]

The implications of Wright's thought is that if there is no
father present in the family, it is important that there be a third
consistent object so that the child can identify with it outside the
symbiotic union.

The child feels drawn to the allure of the exclusive symbiotic
dyad. The father is found in the world and therefore becomes
associated with the world-other-than-mother in the beginning.

The child can lose the mother and find the father. The child identifies the father with the world because he is the world-other-than-mother. The following vignette illustrates the role of the father in separation.

Marjorie was an adult patient who described her mother as domineering and overbearing and her father as emotionally absent except for acting as the mother's enforcer. To escape the familial chaos, Marjorie, as a child, withdrew into her room to daydream or read adventure stories. Before falling asleep, she had an ongoing daydream that was serialized like a soap opera. Since the protagonists in the adventure stories were typically boys, she imagined herself to be a boy. In the dream the little boy befriended a man on a wagon train who was either the wagon train leader or the chief cook. The man taught the boy to ride and to start a campfire. The wagon train was attacked by bandits or Indians. The boy acted bravely but was hurt. He ran out to rescue a horse and was injured. The man he had befriended carried him to safety. It was thrilling to be carried. The man praised the boy for his bravery.

Marjorie had an older brother who was allowed much more freedom because he was a boy. She identified herself with the boy in the adventure story to assume the position of her brother and thereby not be so restricted. The man who befriended her represented a good father who would not be absent but would help her to enter the world-other-than-mother and to save her from the mother's retaliation.

THE MATERNAL AND PATERNAL FUNCTIONS AND BUBER'S I–YOU AND I–IT RELATIONSHIPS

Buber (1958) divided human interactions into I–you and I–it relationships. The you was translated from Buber's German *du*, which has an intimate connotation. The I–you relationship refers to a wholehearted genuine encounter, a living mutual dyad between two individuals who accept and enhance each other's being. Ticho (1974) compared Buber's I–you relationship to Winnicott's holding relationship that supports being. Furthermore, the I–you relationship occurs in a space between each participant, as Winnicott's refers to an intermediate or potential space for transitional objects, play, and creativity. Both Buber's I–you relationship and Winnicott's holding relationship are an expression of the maternal function that provides an authentic sense of being. The I–it relationship, on the other hand, is analytic, dissecting, detached in which the individuals relate to one another as objects, objectively, and not fully as persons. It is the I–it relationship that is concerned with knowledge and analyzing the whole object into its constituent parts.

Buber felt that, in its most primitive form, the individual is involved in the I–it relationship as a part person rather than a whole person. He emphasized that the I–you and the I–it mode have their place and that the human being could not function in the world without both. However, if the individual functioned only on the basis of the I–it relationship, he would not be fully human. The I–it relationship and Winnicott's notion of doing are both expressions of the paternal function.

Winnicott stated that for doing to be authentic and real and not the expression of a false self-system, it must rest on a genuine foundation of being. Winnicott described doing as an expression of the male element of the personality, being as an expression of the female element of the personality. As doing is based on being, the paternal function is based on the maternal function.

Interpreting is an I–it function based upon analyzing clinical phenomena into their constitutive parts. Holding is an I–you function based upon supporting the patient in an authentic sense of being. Following the historical development of psychoanalysis, this chapter focuses on the I–it function of interpretation. The I–you function of holding will be discussed in a later chapter. The discovery of holding occurred later in the historical evolution of psychoanalytic theory although the holding maternal function addresses earlier phases of development than the later interpretive paternal function.

2

KARL ABRAHAM
AND CLASSICAL
OBJECT RELATIONS
INTERPRETATION

Melanie Klein was analyzed by Karl Abraham in Germany. (Her first analyst was Sandor Ferenczi in Budapest, who originated the maternal mode of therapy and whose work will be discussed at length in a later chapter.) Abraham, who was one of the original analysts in the classical tradition, made important theoretical and clinical contributions to what would later be termed object relations theory. Although both Klein and Ronald Fairbairn fully acknowledged Abraham's influence, his contributions are rarely recognized in the current object relations literature. His pioneering paper "A Short Study in the Development of the Libido, Viewed in the Light of Mental Disorders" (Abraham 1924) elaborated on the psychosexual stages and described the development of internalized objects associated with each phase. This paper influenced Klein in the discovery of the depressive position and Fairbairn in his theory of psychopathology. Abraham's clinical paper "A Particular Form of Neurotic Resistance against the Psychoanalytic Method" (1919) was among the first discussions on the difficulties of treating patients diagnosed as narcissistic personality disorders. Abraham was mostly known for his vivid and astute clinical case descriptions and for clear elaboration of classical theory.

INTERPRETING THE LOSS OF
INTERNAL OBJECTS

Freud (1917) stated that in normal mourning the person is conscious of the object loss, whereas in melancholia or depression the
loss may be entirely unconscious. It will be recalled that Freud
found that the depressive patient directed self-reproaches against a
lost love object that the ego had incorporated and identified with.
Abraham (1924) elaborated on the nature of the unconscious loss
that preceded incorporation. He stated that the depressive often
experienced the loss of the love object through the fantasy of anal
expulsion. In other words, the internal object is fantasized as feces
and expelled as such. Abraham believed that many neurotic individuals or depressed individuals react in an anal way to loss by
developing constipation or diarrhea. Constipation is an unconscious effort to retain the object, and diarrhea signifies the expulsion
of the object.

At this point, I will introduce a brief clinical vignette to
illustrate this idea. An 8-year-old child was removed from his
abusive and neglectful family to live in a foster home. After several
months he became attached to the foster family, who provided
good care and security. The courts deemed his natural family was
again able to care for him, so the boy had to leave the foster family
and return to the natural family. He reacted neither sadly nor
angrily. His therapist asked how he felt about the change and he
replied, "When you have to go, you have to go."

Shortly thereafter, the child developed encopresis, which was
characterized by the excessive holding of his bowels and then the
loss of control. Abraham's theory suggests that the child enacted his
conflict about loss through the holding on or evacuating of his
feces. Thus feces stood for the lost object.

Abraham suggested that the expulsion of the object as feces is
experienced in unconscious fantasy as the destruction of the object.
The evacuated feces is understood to be a carcass. The evacuated
object has been destroyed or killed. Abraham (1924) described a
patient who suffered the loss of a significant other and then experienced compulsive thoughts about eating excrement that was lying
about in the street. The expulsion of the object leaves the patient

feeling empty and isolated so that there is a wish to eat the carcass to bring it back to life.

A patient I treated constantly complained of overeating junk food. It made her feel "full of shit." At other times she complained of never achieving her goals. She said, "I say I'm going to do something but never do it. I'm full of shit." I noticed that toward the end of each session, she became detached and did not seem to pay attention to our dialogue. When I explored this, she became aware that toward the end of each session, she had the feeling that I, the therapist, was full of shit and this analysis was worthless. Exploring the binging more carefully, I learned that she binged the most following our session. Thus I interpreted, "As you are about to leave, the pain of separation results in your turning me and the analysis into shit. Your detachment signifies the evacuation of the analyst and our relationship as a piece of shit. You leave feeling empty and isolated, that you have destroyed me and the analysis so that you binge on junk food to take back in the shit. You then come in complaining that you are full of shit, that weighs you down, that you never get anything done or do what you plan. Thus the shit you complain about being full of is actually me."

I recalled another patient who was chronically angry at everyone in her life. She complained of having to take "crap" from everyone she knew. She always said, "Everyone feeds me a lot of crap and I choke on it." Abraham's theory suggests that in chronic anger, the patient is expelling objects; feeling empty, she takes them in as crap. She then is choking on her own bad objects.

Abraham (1924) noted that the depressive patient experienced obsessive-compulsive symptoms at intervals between depressive episodes. He believed that the obsessive-compulsive symptoms reflected a struggle to retain the object and the depression reflected the experience of losing the object. The obsessive-compulsive neurotic who did not become depressed was therefore successful in the struggle to retain the object. Abraham looked at the obsessive-compulsive efforts to order, to control everything and everyone, to possess and collect, to never throw anything away as reflecting the struggle to retain the internal object.

Abraham (1924) explained the nature of these internal objects in terms of the organically determined development of the libidinal aim of the erotogenic zone. He divided each phase in two. Thus there was a preambivalent and ambivalent oral phase, an anal expulsive and anal retentive phase, and a phallic and genital phase. He introduced the idea of the internalization of the object as an aspect of childhood development. In the preambivalent oral phase, the libidinal aim was the incorporation of the breast. This resulted in an internal breast that was divided into good and bad, the good breast cathected by libido, the bad breast by aggression. In accord with the constitutional development of anality, the internal breast was transformed into feces. In the earlier anal phase, the instinctual aim, marked by the heightening of aggression, was the expulsion of the object. The threat of object loss gave rise to an upsurge of libido in the interest of retaining the object. The phallus was also initially fantasized as a part-object and incorporated in the same mode of earlier objects, often in the oral mode pointing to its ancestry of the breast. Abraham described the natural development of the internal part-object: breast, feces, and phallus. The part-objects were experienced by the child in accord with the quality and intensity of the instinctual drive. Thus part-objects could be experienced as precious, treasured, powerful, persecutory, or poisonous, depending on whether they were cathected with libido or aggression.

Abraham found that the anal phase, especially the capacity to retain the object in the face of the destructive urge to expel and destroy it, was a dividing line for the neurosis and psychosis. His viewpoint anticipates current object relations theory in suggesting that the conserving of an internal object (object constancy) is a precondition for averting the psychoses. Furthermore, his dividing line of anality points to the current theory of the borderline who is fixated at the rapprochement stage, the height of anality, in a struggle to retain or expel the object.

Abraham's view remained classical in that he attributed the capacity to retain the object as determined by the quality or strength of the instinctual drive. In the case of the classically depressed patient, the libidinal need of the preambivalent oral phase was innately overly intense giving rise to greater than usual frustration and thereby increasing oral and anal sadism which thereby resulted in the loss of the object. If the anal sadistic drive was not overwhelming, the drive to evacuate the object gave rise to the libidinally determined obsessive-compulsive effort to retain and control the object as described earlier.

I do not accept Abraham's metapsychology. His view remains classical in that the object is a means to an end serving the instinctual impulse tension-reducing goal. However, his views remain clinically important. The infant, unable to tolerate the gap of separateness between itself and the mother, tends to fill this empty core with internal objects. I am not speaking here of a positive recollected image of the mother that can be reinforced by a transitional object and later symbol formation, the ideal situation described by Wright. Rather, I am referring to the lack of a positive recollected experience of the mother that must therefore be filled with concrete things. The incorporation of internal part-objects is felt to be concrete because they are fantasized in terms of breast, feces, and phallus. When the boy described earlier lost the good foster family, he fantasized that he internalized them so as not to need the external objects. The internal object is what Sartre (1940) referred to as "the presence of an absence" (p. 104). This painful absence can be concretized by fantasizing it to be feces. Thus feces becomes a concrete presence to fill the void. This process can then be continued by having concrete things in the external world signify feces, which in turn signifies the painful presence of an absence. John Bowlby pointed to this process in describing children who have lost a parent becoming resigned and low-keyed and shifting their interest from people to nonhuman things. Jean-Paul Sartre (1943) discusses in phenomenological terms how the experience of an inner void gives rise to natural needs to acquire and to possess, to create a sense of substantiality.

THE TIMING OF INTERPRETATION

In "A Particular Form of Neurotic Resistance against the Psycho-analytic Method" Abraham (1919) described a group of patients who keep up seemingly uninterrupted free associations. Their associations, however, are not really free, do not allow for any interruptions by the therapist and are subject to extensive censorship by the ego. The patients differ from other patients who manifest resistances to free associating by arguing that "nothing occurred" to them. In fact, they often express a superabundance of associations, but their very willingness and extraordinarily eager attitude hide their resistance. They may readily tell their dreams but focus on manifest content and can only recognize what they already know. They only discuss what is ego syntonic. Abraham remarked that these patients are especially sensitive to an injury of self-love. They tend to be easily humiliated by interpretations and are on their guard against such humiliation. The patients rarely seek an analysis to alleviate suffering but rather hope that analysis will advance them to a higher level of enlightenment or intellect so that they will be superior to others or can assist in the writing of an autobiography or a new philosophy. In this paper, Abraham wrote, probably for the first time in the history of psychoanalysis, of the difficult resistances of patients who are today diagnosed as narcissistic personalities. He stated that these patients usually have obsessive-compulsive personalities but are unusually prone to narcissistic injury by the process of psychoanalysis. Thus he referred to them as narcissistic neurotics.

Such patients often want to do all of the analysis by themselves. Instead of developing a positive transference, they tend to identify with the therapist. They typically do much of the analysis on their own, at intervals between sessions, a process often termed autoanalysis. They complain of making little progress during analysis and having to work for many hours alone. Abraham explained this phenomenon in terms of narcissistic gratification, a form of daydreaming substitutive of masturbation, and a revolt against the therapist as father. These patients also have pronounced anal sadistic trends, and the process of free association is unconsciously equated with emptying the bowels. Abraham felt that they take pride when, where, whether, and how much they let go of unconscious material.

Abraham recommended interpreting the nature of the resistances at the beginning of the treatment. There is an emphasis on focusing on the difficulties of the treatment, especially the narcissism in all its forms and the revolt against the father in the transference. Abraham (1920) also emphasized interpreting the sadistic significance of defecation. Diarrhea is viewed as a somatic expression of rage. Abraham pointed out that the enraged infant exhibits the same facial expressions, gestures, and bodily movements when it moves its bowels. Some patients react to an event that excites rage with an attack of diarrhea. An evacuation of the bowels can therefore offer to the unconscious of the patient a displaced avenue to express rage. Abraham introduced a theoretical view here that strongly influenced Melanie Klein, that the functions of the bladder and bowel could be in the service of sadism and that urine and flatus are "instruments of a sadistic attack" (p. 319). He interpreted that the patient resisting free association defends against a sadistic attack of the analysis and that free associations were equivalent to diarrhea, which was equated with destroying the object.

His interpretations, of course, were based on clinical material. For instance, a female patient of Abraham's dreamed of sitting in a basket chair near a big lake. A great gust of wind gave rise to a huge wave that engulfed a boat. The patient's father and brother were in the boat. The people swimming in the lake were also drowned. Only one woman swam to the patient, who had little sympathy and did not help her. Abraham interpreted as follows. The German word *stuhl* meant both chair and feces. The basket chair the patient sat on symbolized her stool, or feces. The wind and water that engulfed and drowned her father, brother, and the woman (who stood for her mother) symbolized flatus and urine. Thus the dreamer's family was exterminated by wind and water. The detachment through which she viewed the catastrophe aroused Abraham's suspicion that she herself was the cause of the disaster.

Abraham believed that the patient's resistance to free expression was due to the fear of object loss resulting from sadism. He emphasized that envy was an important factor in the resistance of the narcissistic patient. He interpreted that the patient must devalue and reject the good interpretations of the analyst father. There was also an inability to accept the oedipal parents and their exclusive space. The patient attempts to destroy the oedipal parents through fantasized sadistic attacks of urine and feces. As his earlier paper, "A Short Study on the Development of the Libido" (1924), showed, Abraham also was increasingly aware of the patient's ambivalence toward the preoedipal internal object. His interpretations thus were directed at effecting separation with the preoedipal mother and the parental couple. Symptoms were viewed as disguising the sadism toward objects that resulted in object loss. Abraham pointed the way for Melanie Klein and later object relations therapists to direct interpretations with increasing precision to effect separation from the symbiotic mother.

3

MELANIE KLEIN AND THE INTERPRETATION OF PRIMITIVE PHANTASY

Melanie Klein began her work with children in the 1920s. She originated the play technique. By using the child's play in all its forms—dolls, puppets, drawings, and so on—she gained direct access to the unconscious of the child. The phantasy life of the preoedipal period was made available and the child became increasingly able to verbalize its conflicts. Through this purely psychoanalytic technique, she developed her own theoretical views about the prevalence of the defenses of projection, introjection, splitting, devaluation, and idealization in the first years of life. She showed that introjection resulted in the building up of a complex world of internal objects. The Kleinian technique for adult patients was based on her theoretical views.

Hanna Segal (1981) states that the formal setting in Kleinian technique is identical to that of classical analysis. The patient is seen five times a week for fifty-minute sessions, the couch and analyst's chair are in the classical position, the patient is asked to free associate, and the analyst provides interpretations. In fact, the Kleinian analyst often adheres to the interpretive method even more strictly than the classical technique recommends, rejecting all judgment, advice, reassurance, support, and encouragement. Nevertheless, the Kleinian method can be said to mark an evolutionary departure from the classical technique in the nature of the interpretations given to the patient (Segal 1981). Whereas the classical technique provides interpretation directed toward separation from the oedipal mother, the Kleinian technique focused on separation from the preoedipal mother.

THE INTERPRETATION OF PHANTASY

Melanie Klein wrote her seminal paper "A Contribution to the Psychogenesis of Manic Depressive States" in 1935. She acknowledged her indebtedness to Karl Abraham, especially to the influence of the papers discussed in the preceding chapter, and endeavored to make explicit what was only implicit in his work. In Abraham's view, depressive pathology involved ambivalence toward an internal object and regression to an oral fixation, but normal mourning involved only the loss of an external object. In the Kleinian view, ambivalence toward an internal object and associated depressive anxieties were a normal position in development. Klein showed that internal objects are an inherent aspect of phantasy. It is therefore essential to understand her concept of phantasy in order to discuss her technical approach.

    For Klein, unconscious phantasy is a direct derivative of the instincts and the conflict between them. Susan Isaacs (1948) defined phantasy as "the mental correlate of the instincts," (p. 9) or the psychic equivalent of the instincts. Segal (1981) stated, "In the infant's omnipotent world, instincts express themselves as the phantasy of their fulfillment" (p. 5). Unconscious phantasy is therefore the mental representation of the instinctual impulse. For Klein, the infant is endowed with the tendency of phantasizing at birth. The object is initially affective because it derives from the infant's first sensations of pleasure and pain. Hinshelwood (1989) adds that "an unconscious phantasy is a belief in a concretely felt object" (p. 34). An instinctual drive gives rise to a somatic sensation that evokes a mental experience. This is interpreted as a relationship to an object that is evoking the pleasant or unpleasant sensation. If pleasant, it is felt as the presence of a good object, if unpleasant, as caused by a bad object. For instance, hunger, a gnawing in the stomach, is felt as a bad object. Unpleasant experience is felt by the infant as the pain of dying or annihilation. The hunger is therefore projected onto the external object, and the outer object is now perceived as hungry or devouring. The infant may internalize the bad, devouring object in order to control it. Thus through projective identification, the infant's own hunger, greed, or envy is encased in the object.

In the Kleinian view, phantasy is primitive, constantly active, and coloring and interplaying with external reality. This view results in a theory of the person living in two worlds at the same time, an inner psychic world, which is expressed through phantasy, and an outer material world. The ego relates with both the internal and external object worlds. The earliest object relationships with significant others enter into one's psychic life and become structures of the personality, and it is impossible to keep the two worlds of inner and outer reality completely apart. Events in the outer world stir up relationships with deeply buried internal objects, and feelings toward inner objects color relationships with outer objects.

Klein's views of phantasy directly affect technique. The patient's material may seem indisputably concerned with external facts, but there may be an element of unconscious phantasy contained in facts. For instance, if a patient remarks that it is nasty, cold, and dreary outside, the analyst may wonder if the patient complains that the analyst is nasty, cold and dreary, thereby causing the patient to feel depressed. Kleinian analysts believe that the analyst is the central figure in the patient's phantasy world in that the analyst is believed to be identified with a significant internal object of the patient.

The following vignette illustrates the technique of interpreting the patient's living in two worlds at the same time. An adult female patient arrived for her second therapy session. She briefly described the events of the week and then wondered what she might discuss for this session. I told her that she could discuss whatever came to mind. It was the day that President Bush became ill during his trip to Japan. She said, "What do you think about what happened to George Bush today?"

I recounted the facts that I had heard about the incident and asked what she thought. She said, "I felt terrible for him. I learned of it after it became known that he was only ill with the flu, but I still felt terrible. I like Bush. I think that he is a man with good intentions. I believe he went to Japan to try to help people here, but it went wrong. It's a bad break for him.''

My response was aimed at identifying the element of unconscious phantasy contained in her remarks about the president's trip. I said, "The way we feel when something like this occurs may tell us something about ourselves as well as the situation. Our own history and life events color how we understand the circumstances around us. The president is often felt to be a parental figure for the country because of his position of authority and leadership. When something happens to a president our interpretation of the events may have something to do with how we would feel if something happened to our own parents or be related to our feelings about them. This is not speaking to the truth or falseness of the interpretation itself. George Bush may happen to be as well intentioned as you believe, or his intentions may be entirely different. This I cannot comment on, nor is it relevant for us. Our concern is what you make of such an event based on your particular history, not the event itself.''

The patient replied that she thought she knew what I meant. She recalled how upset people were when John Kennedy was assassinated. It was as if the country lost its parent. She said, "But my father isn't at all like George Bush. Bush is the type of father I wish I had. My father is a gambler.'' She described several stories in which her father gambled away the family's money and fought with her mother. She added, "It wasn't that he didn't care about us. He told himself he would win and we would all be happy. He was a good man and had good intentions, but he had bad luck and couldn't control himself.'' She realized that she characterized her father in the same terms with which she had earlier described George Bush, a good man with good intentions. She said she felt the same way over the incident of the Russian coup. She thought of Gorbachev as a good man with good intentions that went wrong. She cried when the coup occurred. She thought of Gorbachev as a Santa Claus. She said, "I see Bush and Gorbachev as gamblers like my father. Bush gambled on Japan and Gorbachev gambled on perestroika.''

Further along in her treatment, the question might be raised as to whether she defends against anger at her father by insisting on his good intentions.

ANXIETY AND DEFENSES

The Kleinian technique involves providing interpretations that are directed at the level at which anxiety occurs. Anxiety is believed to be active in association with phantasy. The Kleinian analyst often interprets material earlier and more directly than the classical analyst. Thus a severely disturbed patient acting in a first session as if he were frightened by the analyst may be told that he projects his aggression onto the analyst and therefore fears him. The interpretation is believed to lessen the patient's persecutory anxieties and thereby allow him to remain in the session. Kleinians believe that interpretations should provide understanding of psychotic defenses and the anxieties that give rise to them. Interpretations are directed at content as well as the defenses against it. Defenses are not viewed as mechanisms but rather as facets of phantasy life. For instance, projection and introjection are based on primitive phantasies of incorporation and ejection. The Kleinian analyst may interpret repression as the manifestation of a phantasy of dams built inside the body holding back a flood or denial as a phantasy of objects that are annihilated. There is no interpretation of mechanisms but rather of phantasies contained in mechanisms.

THE PARANOID-SCHIZOID POSITION

Melanie Klein (1935, 1946) described two phases of the oral stage that are central to her theory and technique: the paranoid-schizoid and depressive positions. These correspond roughly to Abraham's preambivalent and ambivalent oral phases. Klein viewed them as innately programmed, automatic, and inevitable. In my view, the outcomes of these phases depend on the quality of early object relationships, not innate programming. I am in agreement with Kenneth Wright that they remain useful ideas if they are thought about as two modes of organizations or structuring of psychic functions. The earlier paranoid-schizoid position evolves into the depressive position.

According to Klein (1946), in the paranoid-schizoid position the infant has no concept of a whole person but is related to part-objects or simpler structures as they function independently of one another. The whole object is split into an idealized and persecutory object, and the pervasive anxiety is persecutory, the fear of forces destroying the ideal self and the ideal object. The infant attempts to keep apart the ideal and persecutory objects in order to protect the ideal object. Splitting, introjection, projection, and denial are the active mechanisms of defense. The Kleinian technique focuses on interpreting persecutory objects and defenses against them. If the relationship to the analyst is idealized, it is especially important to interpret any "bad" figures in the patient's life who may be containing split-off bad aspects of the patient or analyst.

A female patient with an idealizing transference entered the analyst's office and said, "When you buzzed me into the building another woman walked in behind me." She laughed and added, "Maybe she's an ax-murderess."

The analyst immediately interpreted that the ax-murderess was a split-off denied aspect of the patient's aggression, but the patient strongly rejected the interpretation. It would have been more effective for the analyst to refrain from interpretation and await the material to follow. It is likely that there would have been enough hints of conflict over aggression for the therapist to relate the conflictual material to the patient's opening remarks.

Projection and projective identification are central defenses of the paranoid-schizoid position. In both projection and projective identification, the ego rids itself of unwanted parts by phantasizing that they are projected onto the other. In projective identification, there is the additional factor that the projected or encased part of the self is phantasized to be controlling the other it is encased within. Analysts who focus on interpersonal relationships as well as internal object relationships emphasize that through projective identification, the patient actually pressures the other to feel the effect of the projected part.

The following example illustrates the distinction between

projection and projective identification. A patient denied any dependence or feelings of distress as the time approached for the therapist's vacation. However, the patient complained that her daughter was becoming needy, demanding, and infantile. The therapist interpreted projection by stating that the daughter represented the needy, infantile, demanding side of the patient, who was indeed upset by the therapist's vacation. The therapist could interpret projective identification by adding that the patient phantasized putting the demanding, infantile, needy part of herself into the daughter and thereby controlling it.

Melanie Klein (1946) drew on Freud's speculative ideas of a life and death instinct to explain the paranoid–schizoid position. She was among the first to develop a psychodynamic analysis of the development of aggression. She demonstrated how aggression remained of crucial importance in psychic life, created anxiety and, through projection and introjection, was a major factor in severe pathologies. For Klein, anxiety is the perception of a death instinct or primary masochism that threatens the infant with annihilation. It is for this reason that aggression initially is projected into the mother, thereby giving rise to the paranoid–schizoid position. Klein is to be credited for her close attention to the postnatal development of aggression, although she attributed aggression predominantly to an innate death instinct and primary sadism and not to the ill effects of environmental frustration or bad objects. As Guntrip (1961) pointed out, Klein's belief in the death instinct obscured the fact that her own work implied that aggression may be a reactive development to the ill effects of a bad environment or bad objects that are internalized. As the next chapter illustrates, Ronald Fairbairn contended that Klein's work pointed to an equal emphasis on parental impact and on the subjective development of the bad object situation for the child, an area neglected by Klein because of her focus on the death instinct and innate sadism.

Although I do not accept Klein's metapsychology nor her theory of the death instinct as the origin of aggression, I nevertheless believe that her views on aggression have considerable clinical importance. Klein's theory amounted to a reorientation of psychoanalysis centering on aggression as opposed to libido as the crucial factor in severe pathology. One need not accept Klein's metapsychology of the origins of aggression to realize that our own aggression toward others may color our view of them or give rise to a fear of retaliation. Klein's theory of projective identification provides the therapist with the framework to interpret the patient projection of rage onto external objects.

CLINICAL EXAMPLES

A patient consistently arrived late for her sessions. When the therapist questioned why the patient was late or remarked on the patient's ambivalence about coming, the patient replied that the therapist must be angry that she was late. The therapist interpreted that the patient believed that the therapist is angry because she herself is angry and therefore expects the therapist to be angry and to retaliate. The therapist added that the patient is late in the first place because she is angry. The therapist should be careful to explain that he is not saying the patient is purposefully coming late to provoke the therapist's anger. Rather, the patient is unconscious of her anger and perceives it as coming from the therapist. This is an interpretation of a projection. If the therapist wished to interpret projective identification, he would add that the patient attempts to rid herself of her anger by putting it into the therapist and making the therapist feel as she does. In this way she could feel that she controls the therapist and avoid feeling that the therapist is in control. This second interpretation is more challenging than the first and should not be given unless the patient has a very good understanding of psychic processes and a strong rapport with the therapist and is unlikely to feel attacked. In making this interpretation the emphasis should be on the patient's need to be rid of difficult feelings by having the therapist feel them as opposed to saying that the patient tries to provoke the therapist.

A married male patient prone to attacks of rage repeatedly described how his wife was critical, complaining, and provoking and how he had no recourse but to attack in self-defense. He described the various issues for which his wife picked on him and felt that it was unfair for her to injure him this way. The therapist acknowledged that it did sound as if his wife could be overly critical, but that the patient reacted as if severely attacked. This may be because he felt that what she picked on him for was terrible, which made him angry at himself. Since he felt that these things about himself were terrible, he must have believed that his wife felt this way too and that his rage at himself was really directed at her.

A female patient's husband suffered a sudden heart attack. For a few weeks he was in critical condition. As she became more assured of his survival, she became increasingly fearful of potential muggers and other criminals on the street. She was also hypersensitive to any remarks made by friends, relatives, or the hospital staff, as she was quick to feel attacked. The therapist interpreted that her husband's illness terrified her. As it became more likely that he would survive, she became angry at him for being ill and for frightening her. She did not allow herself to be angry at him because she still feared losing him. Instead, she projected her anger onto the world and perceived it as more dangerous and attacking. Furthermore, when she felt criticized by someone, she felt justified in her anger and therefore could allow its expression through the displacement.

THE DEPRESSIVE POSITION

Klein (1935) found that the depressive organization is a more integrated structure in which part-objects came together into the whole mother. The dilemma is that the attacked object is identical to the object that is loved; guilt, concern, and reparation emerge as the functions of the new organization. In systems theory, these are new controlling functions of the organization (Wright 1991b). In the paranoid-schizoid position, the infant fears being destroyed by its persecutors. In the depressive position, it fears its own aggression will destroy the good object. Because it experiences phantasy as omnipotent, the infant experiences its aggression as destroying the object. The mother's absence may be thought of as a death. In states of depressive anxiety and mourning, it believes not only that the external object is lost but also that the internal mother is destroyed.

Efforts at reparation signify the libidinal wish to repair the internal object.

I see a close correspondence between Klein's theory of the depressive position and Mahler's concept of the rapprochement subphase of separation–individuation. Mahler (1975) suggested that the toddler separates with aggression. Wishing to separate, the toddler phantasizes that the mother feels abandoned and expects that she will retaliate by abandoning him. The child therefore returns to the mother with a gift from its adventures in order to reconnect. Klein's description of the depressive position is the unconscious phantasy associated with the experience of rapprochement. The child's aggressive separation is felt to injure her. The mother phantasized as injured is experienced consciously as feeling abandoned. The absence of the mother is unconsciously phantasized as the destruction of the mother. Klein noted that the infant dreads retaliation by the injured or destroyed object. The toddler's fear that the object will never return and thus has abandoned him is the conscious experience of the destroyed object's retaliation. Rapprochement is therefore the conscious expression of the child's unconscious efforts to repair the injured object. Klein posited the depressive position at 6 months, whereas Mahler identified rapprochement at around 18 months. This discrepancy in ages is less of a problem if the depressive position and rapprochement are viewed not as fixed and programmed stages of development but rather as modes of organizing experience. It is likely that throughout life the individual oscillates, to varying degrees, between the paranoid-schizoid and depressive positions, although the latter would be deemed the more advanced, differentiated, and complex structure.

THE MANIC DEFENSE

The depressive position is central to development and to psychopathology in Kleinian theory. Her technique focuses on the interpretation of paranoid-schizoid phenomena as a depressive regression from depressive anxiety. The manic defense is characterized by splitting, idealization, devaluation, denial, and projective identification, the defense mechanisms characterizing the paranoid-schizoid position. For Klein (1946), the paranoid-schizoid position is therefore utilized defensively to retreat from the conflicts of the depressive position. Klein referred to this defensive use of paranoid-schizoid defenses as the manic defense. It is the pain of object loss that mobilizes the manic defenses. The infant's recognition of the mother as a whole object that gratifies and frustrates gives rise to ambivalence, the fear of loss and associated guilt. It is primarily the experience of separation and loss that the infant or patient tries to deny through the manic defense. There may be denial of the object as a whole, of dependence on the object, or of the importance of the object. There is typically a phantasy of omnipotent control or triumph over the object replacing depressive feelings of loss.

In the August 12, 1992, issue of *The Manchester Guardian* a story appeared about a 12-year-old boy whose mother suffered a stroke that left her paralyzed. As she lay dying, the boy went on a spending spree for several days, buying his friends whatever they wished. The authorities were horrified that he never called for help, instead leaving his mother paralyzed on the floor of their apartment. However, when a neighbor found her and called the authorities, the boy broke down and cried as the ambulance arrived and carried off his mother.

In Kleinian terms, the boy may have denied the loss by his indifference and manic spending spree. Buying his friends whatever they wanted may have been an effort at omnipotently controlling the internal object projected onto them, thereby serving the denial of loss. The denial finally dissipated when the boy broke down at the sight of the authorities arriving to help his ailing mother.

Segal (1981) points out that the manic defense results in a vicious cycle. The original aggression toward the object leads to depression. The manic defenses deny the depression but prevent a working through of the depressive position. The effort at omnipotent control, triumph, and contempt for the object reflects a further attack on the object. Kleinian analysts look for the depression underlying manic material and mania underlying depressive material.

As Freud interpreted the patient's resistances against separation from the oedipal mother, Klein focused on separation from the preoedipal mother. The Kleinians focus on the interpretation of the manic defense to uncover the denial of loss, separateness, and mourning. As Susan Kavaler-Adler (1992) has pointed out, the patient's experience of mourning for the lost objects in the transference is an essential aspect of analysis. I have mostly emphasized the interpretive aspects of the Kleinian technique, but the analyst also holds the patient through the mourning process. Kavaler-Adler believes that the patient's erotic transference, extreme dependence, and aggression may all be related to mourning and loss.

The Kleinian technique of interpretation of the defenses against dependence aims to uncover the patient's denial of loss and separateness. By acknowledging this dependence, the patient becomes aware of object loss and separateness. The vulnerability of dependence results in rage at the object, the threat of object loss, guilt, and depression. The denial of the importance of the object in the manic defense serves to avoid the pain of separation. Thus, when Melanie Klein attempted to interpret the patient's defenses against dependence in the transference, she did not conceptualize dependence as having value for its own sake as a corrective emotional experience for past deficit. This idea would have to wait for the work of Fairbairn, Balint, and Winnicott. Rather, Klein was pointing her patients toward the experience of separateness, object loss, mourning, aggression, and guilt.

The following clinical vignettes illustrate the manic defense.

Case 1

A middle-aged female patient of mine was in analysis for four years. I was about to go away for a summer vacation, but the patient denied any feelings of loss or anger. She complained about feeling rejected by various persons in her life but denied that she could be displacing feeling rejected by my impending departure.

The patient reported a puzzling dream shortly thereafter. She dreamed that she was at work and colleagues from a previous job continually called to leave word that a supportive friend she had not seen for years had died in a car crash. The patient felt indifferent, then rationalized that she was not affected by the loss because the friend had not been a part of her life for many years. Her first association was that the reason she gave for not being upset by the death—that the friend had not played any part in her life for many years—could also prompt a question as to why she should dream of this friend at all. Another puzzling factor was that the colleagues at her former job who informed her of the loss actually could never have known about the death, since she had not met the friend at the job but rather years before at school. In fact, they had had no mutual acquaintances who could have known this information.

I remarked that she dreamed of the loss of a supportive old friend who played no part in her life for many years and that there was no one in her life who knew both her and the friend and could inform her if anything happened to the friend. However, in the dream she was notified by colleagues at a former job of the death of the friend. This only served to draw to her attention that she and the friend actually had no mutual acquaintances, so the persons who informed her, in fact, would be unable to do so. She acknowledged that this was the gist of the dream and her associations about it. I then asked in what other situation in her life were there no mutual acquaintances, no one who could inform her if something happened to a supportive friend. She thought about this for a moment and could think of no other situation that fit this description. She suddenly became aware that the situation applied to her and me— that we knew no one in common and that if anything were to happen to me there would be no one who could inform her. She knew enough about dream interpretation to be aware that a supportive friend who played no part in her current life could easily be a symbol of a "supportive friend" who did play a part in her current life. I then pointed out that in the dream the old supportive friend was killed in a car crash—he was traveling somewhere—and I was about to travel somewhere on vacation. Thus it became apparent that she was unconsciously angry at me for going on vacation, so she killed me off as the supportive friend. The manic defense was demonstrated in her seeming indifference to the loss and her hypersensitivity to rejection by her friends, all of whom she was trying to control to avoid the repressed feelings of loss. It was her very need to control the friends that made her hypersensitive to feeling rejected by them.

Case 2

An 8-year-old child who had been severely deprived and abused came to me for therapy. At first, she timidly explored the office, showing interest in the dirt in a flower pot and the water faucet. Once she became comfortable, she attacked the office. She took the dirt from the pot, spreading it across the play table and floor. As she dirtied the office, she looked to see my reaction. She sprinkled water over the play table, dirt, and toys. She muddied the furniture. She then became anxious and cleaned up. The efforts to clean became urgent, and the cleaning was done with so much energy and effort that it resulted in further wrecking. She scrubbed the play table with so much water that she flooded the area. She attempted to fix a toy until she broke it.

For Melanie Klein, the working through of the depressive position is based on the capacity to make reparation. The playroom and I represented the internal mother. She attacked the object by her destruction of the room. Klein points out that the very young child experiences such bodily expressions of rage as wetting and soiling as phantasies of attacking the parental object. Thus, in Kleinian terms, the dirt, mud, and water symbolized feces and urine, instruments of her aggression; she attacked the object with her feces and urine. The attack led to a fear of object loss, so that she looked at me to make sure that I would not retaliate or abandon her. She attempted to make reparation with the cleaning, but her capacity was weak and reparation became further destruction. Thus there was a manic guilt to the reparative effort. By the end of the session the child refused to leave, omnipotently saying she could do whatever she pleased.

Over the summer I visited her at a camp for emotionally disturbed children. She boasted to her bunkmates of how she messed up my office and I allowed her to do whatever she pleased. It was only gradually, over many months of treatment, that her efforts to clean and repair became less urgent and more constructive. I rarely provided interpretations except for remarking that it was difficult for her to leave at the end of the hour. Instead, I tolerated her acting out and set limits only if she risked hurting herself or irreparably destroying something. The concern here is not so much for the item destroyed but rather for the anxiety produced in the child. The child sees that her constructive, libidinal capacity is not strong enough to offset her destructive tendencies.

ENVY AND THE IDEAL OBJECT

With the publication of *Envy and Gratitude* (1957) Klein devoted increasing attention to paranoid-schizoid phenomena. She emphasized the importance of envy for personality development. She described envy as occurring in a dyadic relationship toward a part-object possessing an attribute that the subject lacked. In contrast, jealousy is felt toward a whole object in a triadic relationship. Klein viewed envy as a direct derivative of the death instinct. The infant envies the life-giving, creative and loving aspects of the maternal breast. Underlying envy is the conflict between the life and death instincts. Klein believed that envy played a crucial role in the negative therapeutic reaction. The patient enviously attacks the goodness and creativity of the analyst's interpretations and empathy. Envy may interfere with the normative aspects of splitting during the paranoid-schizoid phase. There is the failure to split the object into an ideal and bad breast. Envy and hate destroy the ideal object. Herbert Rosenfeld (1987) utilized the Kleinian theory of envy in his work with psychosis, destructive narcissism, and substance abuse. On a clinical level, it is possible to dispense with the Kleinian view of the death instinct and innate envy and to combine Fairbairn's theory that aggression is an instinctual reaction to frustration with Klein's views on envy and the ideal object. In a later chapter I will do exactly that, providing a critique of Rosenfeld's theory of destructive narcissism and envy and advancing a new viewpoint from a Klein–Fairbairn outlook.

KERNBERG'S CRITIQUE OF KLEIN

Kernberg (1980) integrated important aspects of Klein's theory into his own views while providing a critique of her theory and tech-

nique. Kernberg agreed with the Kleinians about the pervasiveness
of the primitive defenses in early development and severe personality disorders but criticized them for placing these complex ego
operations in the first months of life. He integrated Klein's views
with the work of Jacobson and Mahler, thereby placing the primitive defenses within an ego psychological developmental timetable.
Whereas Klein viewed the early defenses as active measures to
organize experience, Kernberg emphasized the ego's incapacity to
synthesize opposing qualities of experience (Grotstein 1981). Kernberg agreed with Klein that a central goal of treatment is the
integration of good and bad part-objects (object constancy in ego
psychological terms) and to effect separation from the preoedipal
mother. Kernberg (1975) and Masterson (1976) both emphasize the
paternal function of the therapist as interpreter. Whereas Kleinians
are likely to make interpretations in the language of good and bad
breasts, Kernberg and Masterson are likely to speak of good and
bad self and parental images. Kernberg's language of interpretation
(1975) reflects his views that transference manifestations are not a
direct reliving of early phantasy or experience but rather structured
internalized object relations configurations appreciably distorted
by the primitive defenses. He therefore focuses transference interpretations on here-and-now activations of internalized object relations units. He believes that there must be a significant lessening of
distortion by primitive defenses before the therapist can accurately
reconstruct genetic material. Kernberg has refined Kleinian technique with ego psychological understanding, but his primary therapeutic aim remains that of providing interpretations to effect
separation from the preoedipal mother. There is a holding aspect to
the views of Kernberg and Masterson in that they emphasize the
affective aspect of primitive defenses and the therapist's containment of the patient's released and painful ambivalence as splitting is
resolved.

MODERN KLEINIAN TECHNIQUE: BETTY JOSEPH AND JAMES GROTSTEIN

Kleinian technique has continued to develop, and its contemporary
representatives have addressed or refined some of its earlier short-

comings. Among the most creative and thoughtful of the Kleinian analysts today are Betty Joseph and James Grotstein.

Betty Joseph

Betty Joseph (1986) has recommended that the analyst remain close to the psychic reality of the moment-by-moment interaction of the analysand and analyst during the session. She points out that change is more a process than a state occurring through a continuation of constant, minute shifts and movements. There may be a minute change in the patient's defensive operation and an anxiety-induced return to the status quo. It is important for the analyst to be aware of these minute changes and to interpret the process in the instant of the patient's effort toward change and return to a security operation. A patient may always idealize that analyst. A moment of ambivalence occurs as the patient alludes to anger at the therapist. The patient then rationalizes the analyst's behavior that angered her and returns to the security of idealization. Joseph's recommendation of interpreting shifts in the patient's defensive system focuses on split-off states. The emphasis is on recognizing the patient's unique way of responding to anxieties about relationship. The analyst should refrain from value judgments about the changes being good or bad but instead emphasize that they are the patient's way to cope. Comments are made in terms of the interaction between patient and analyst, and not exclusively in terms of the patient. The therapist attempts to elicit the patient's take on the interaction and how that may affect his capacity to utilize the therapist's interventions.

> *Patient*: I am in conflict as to whether I should make use of your superior knowledge, learning, and intelligence to deal with the problems of my life—get on with the work, so to speak—or whether I should list my complaints about you—that there are things that you say or do that disturb me.
>
> *Therapist*: So there are issues about our interaction. In one way, you think of me as superior and you can make use of this superiority as you see it. But then there is this other issue that what I say or do sometimes disturbs you and interferes with your own capacity to

make use of what you consider as my superior capacity. How does it affect you to think of me as superior for doing this work? How does it affect your feelings about our interaction?

In this way, the therapist endeavors to present the patient's take on the interaction in a way that facilitates further associations concerning envy, competition, and their relationship, if any, to the patient's other complaints about the therapist. The therapist's first step is to address the patient's view of the therapist's superiority and how this affects the patient's feelings about their interaction. The therapist neither confirms nor denies this perception. The therapist will also need to support the patient's thought of putting all of his negative attitudes about the therapist into words before going on with the analysis.

Joseph (1985) believes that interpretations are more likely to lead to change if they are anchored in the transference–countertransference situation. Kleinian analysts often recommend that the therapist immediately and directly interpret the patient's primitive defenses. Joseph suggests that if it is apparent to the therapist that the patient is utilizing projective identification extensively, the therapist should nevertheless refrain from intervening and wait until the patient utilizes the defense in the transference in order to interpret.

A patient described feeling unmotivated to pursue certain goals that she considered useful and to stop certain behaviors she believed were bad for her. She described incidents in which the persons in her life attempted to persuade her to fulfill these aspirations, but she felt pressured and became more resistant. It was the therapist's sense that she utilized projective identification to make the people in her life feel her own conflictual motivation that she should change. The therapist refrained from making this interpretation and instead waited until he felt induced to pressure her to change. He still made no interpretations but instead paid attention to the minute shifts in interaction that prompted him to feel this way. He noticed that when she described putting off something she felt she should do, her tone of voice became subtly challenging. If she described something she felt she should or should not do, she never talked out the reason she believed she should behave in this way, as if she were leaving it to the therapist to begin to lecture her and to say what she left unspoken. The therapist refrained from acting on these induced feelings, and the patient began to ask how she should motivate herself. The therapist interpreted that she wished the therapist could somehow get her going, stimulate her to change. He added that she tried to put into him her own denied wish to change and have him feel the need for her to change. The therapist said, "You want me to feel your need to change so that you can deny that need and the conflict to change." The therapist explained that she tried to rid herself of the need to change not because she was lazy, but because she was afraid to feel the need for change.

This interpretation gradually resulted in the patient's feeling and owning her own conflict. As the wish for change grew, she became more self-destructive. The therapist then interpreted that she had disowned her need for change because another part of her feared and attacked her for it. This internal saboteur was identified with a parental figure that prevented the patient from growing up emotionally and becoming a self-motivated person who could make her own decisions, choices to lead her own life.

Betty Joseph (1985) emphasizes transference as a total situation. Transference is not viewed simply as a literal transfer of feelings toward whole early objects onto the therapist but rather as a total situation—a complex pattern of unconscious feelings and thought, defenses, anxieties, and expectations that the patient takes into the situation.

Joseph (1983) states, "I have stressed the importance of seeing transference as a living relationship in which there is a constant movement and change. I have indicated how everything of importance in the patient's psychic organization based on early and habitual ways of functioning, his fantasies, impulses, defenses and conflicts, will be lived out in some way in the transference" (p. 167).

Joseph's view of transference as a total situation would fit the phenomena described by Jean-Paul Sartre under the concept of "totalization." The patient's level of psychic functioning is totalized in the transference situation. Joseph recommends that the therapist interpret the transference not through details that identify the analyst as a historical whole object but rather as an expression of the patient's total psychic situation.

A patient manifested much clinical evidence of severe conflicts around merger and loss of autonomy. The patient once complained about having to meet with a friend at least once a week. He felt that the friend was demanding, dependent, and smothering. The patient was often quite resistant, missing sessions or coming late, but denying any ambivalence about the therapy and attributing the lateness to unavoidable circumstances. The therapist remarked that the patient saw the therapist, as well as the friend, once a week. The therapist suggested that the patient may be afraid of being smothered and feel that the therapist is as demanding on his time and money as the friend. The patient denied any connection between his feelings for the friend and the therapist, insisting that the therapist did not remind him of the friend. Joseph's viewpoint suggests that it was a mistake for the therapist to focus on the detail of the patient seeing the friend and the therapist once weekly or on the therapist reminding the patient of the friend, as if there were a direct transfer of feelings toward a whole object. Rather, it might have been more effective to focus on the total situation: that the patient brings to relationships some expectation or concern that he will be smothered or trapped and lose his autonomy. The therapist might have added that some people more than others may elicit this feeling. It also could have been pointed out to the patient that since the friend is in reality smothering and demanding, the patient is aware of his fear of loss of autonomy. Since the therapist had not acted in this way and did not remind the patient of the friend, the patient is not aware of this fear. As the patient begins to recognize the total situation he brings to the transference, he then wonders whether his anxieties are related to what is going on internally or whether it is a realistic reaction to a threat.

Joseph believes that everything the analyst is or says is likely to be responded to according to the patient's own psychic makeup, rather than the analyst's intentions and the meanings he gives to his interpretations. Joseph is pointing out that the patient also interprets the analyst's interpretation, not in terms of the provision of insight but rather in accord with the patient's total situation. The analyst may interpret splitting or fragmentation and the patient may feel that the analyst is sadistically tearing him to pieces. Therefore, the therapist must closely follow and elicit the patient's reactions and interpretations of the analyst's interpretations.

James Grotstein

As Betty Joseph has refined and elaborated upon Kleinian technique, James Grotstein advances it through his original understanding and creative application of Klein's views.

Grotstein (1981) says that the psychoanalytic treatment of splitting has not achieved the importance it deserves. He points out that Freud's description of splitting in terms of instinctual impulses that were warded off by repression but achieved consciousness is misleading. The motivations of split-off selves are more complex with a life and agenda of their own. Split-off subpersonalities are also intermingled with internalized objects formed by projective identification and subsequent introjection. Split selves act as separate personifications in the same self system. For instance, a split-off addictive state has a motivational support system and agenda of its own undermining the central self state that battles the addiction. Grotstein emphasizes that such split-off self states are critical to an understanding of psychoses, depression, and narcissism. Melanie Klein implicitly conceived of splitting as manifesting separate, dissociated subself states, which Fairbairn later made explicit. The importance of subself states related to internal objects for interpretive techniques will be elaborated on in the next chapter on the work of Fairbairn.

4

RONALD FAIRBAIRN AND THE BRIDGE BETWEEN INTERPRETING AND HOLDING

W. R. D. Fairbairn was greatly indebted to Melanie Klein for the theory of internalized objects. Nevertheless, Fairbairn disagreed with Klein on basic assumptions. Whereas Klein believed that structural differentiation occurred under the internal, disintegrating impact of the death instinct, Fairbairn argued that structural differentiation began under the disturbing influence of bad object relations in actual life. For Klein, anxiety is not an object relations phenomenon but an innate phenomenon due to a tendency to ego disintegration under the impact of the death instinct. Fairbairn also rejected Klein's belief that the infant started off with destructive relations to the breast. He advanced the views of Abraham and Klein to a complete object relations theory. It is this writer's view that Fairbairn provides the most consistent and comprehensive outlook among object relations theorists.

Fairbairn (1958) felt that throughout his major writings he made only the scantest references to implications for psychoanalytic technique. In fact, he acknowledged that his writings could lead to the impression that his contributions left analytic technique unaffected. In a later paper on "The Nature and Aims of Psychoanalytic Treatment" (1958), Fairbairn stated that such an inference would be entirely inaccurate. He maintained that the practice implications of his views were quite radical and far-reaching. At the same time, Fairbairn was a conservative practitioner and believed that the technical implications of his views should be put to the test only gradually and with considerable circumspection to prevent premature, mistaken, or rash changes in practice.

After the introductory words of caution, Fairbairn announced the direction he believed analytic therapy should take. He stated that although interpretation remained an important technique, it was not enough and that the relationship between the patient and analyst provided more than a medium or setting for the interpretation of the transference situation. He said,

> In terms of the object-relations theory of the personality, the disabilities from which the patient suffers represent the effects of unsatisfactory object-relationships in early life and perpetuated in an exaggerated form in inner reality—and if this view is correct, the actual relationship existing between the patient and analyst as persons must be regarded as in itself constituting a therapeutic factor of prime importance. The existence of such a personal relationship in outer reality not only serves the function of providing a means of correcting the distorted relationships which prevail in inner reality and influence the reactions of the patient to outer objects, but provides the patient with an opportunity, denied to him in childhood, to undergo a process of emotional development in the setting of an actual relationship with a reliable and beneficent parental figure. [p. 377]

Fairbairn presented the basis for the therapeutic object relationship as providing a corrective emotional experience. However, his views on the therapeutic value of the patient–therapist relationship are not based solely on humanistic values but on his scientific, theoretical formulations concerning human development. Fairbairn's technique is a combination of a positive object relationship to provide the patient with new opportunities for growth and interpretations aimed at dissolving the bad objects dominating the patient's internal psychic life. This internal bad object world is implied in the various forms of resistance. Fairbairn held that the greatest source of all resistance is the maintenance of the patient's internal world as a closed system. He remarked upon the aims of analytic treatment: to cause breaches in the closed system of the patient's bad internal object world, to promote a "synthesis" of the structures into which the original unitary ego is divided, to reduce infantile dependence, and to lessen the hatred of the original libidinal object.

An implication of Fairbairn's work, which has not been fully appreciated in the literature and was never made explicit by him, is that interpretations that provide a breach in the closed internal world of bad objects allow for the patient to establish and incorporate a good object relationship with the therapist. I believe Fairbairn's work to be so important because it implies that interpretation need not always be antithetical to holding but may allow for holding to occur. Given that his technique is fully based upon his theoretical principles, it is necessary to spell them out.

LIBIDO AS OBJECT SEEKING

Fairbairn (1941) stated that the goal of libido is object seeking. He drew a distinction between object seeking and satisfaction seeking that has informed the work of both Balint and Winnicott (Wright 1991b). In classical theory, the object is the signpost to libidinal pleasure or the reduction of libidinal tension. The object is chosen for its availability. The infant becomes accustomed to achieving gratification with the object and forms an attachment. The infant therefore experiences separation anxiety because loss of the object is associated with loss of pleasure. The infant is originally satisfaction seeking in terms of the breast and orality.

Wright (1991b) points out that the infant is drawn to the changing expressions of the face in the first weeks of life prior to recognition of the human face or specific recognition of the mother's face. Eigen, Spitz, and Winnicott have also remarked on the infant's interest in the mother's face as the earliest evidence of an object relationship. As I (Seinfeld 1991b) pointed out in an earlier publication, Fairbairn states that the infantile ego is originally whole and relates to the mother as a separate unitary object, although in a vague, primitive, affective sense. There is therefore a primary intersubjective relationship between the infant and mother. The infant responds to the mother as a subject in its interest in her changing facial expressions and changing voice, both of which show her alive subjectivity. Wright states that the infant's interest in the mother's face expresses object seeking while its relationship to the breast serves satisfaction seeking. John Sutherland (1989) notes that the baby, while nursing at the breast, "drinks" in the expressions of the mother's face, thereby taking in the good object experience (Scharff 1992). This is a clear example of the Fairbairnian idea that when object relations are good, satisfaction seeking serves object seeking. Satisfaction seeking and object seeking split off when there is a failure in good object relating. However, given that it is inevitable that object relating will, to a degree, be unsatisfactory, there will always be some splitting of satisfaction and object seeking.

OBJECT RELATIONS THEORY AND THE PHILOSOPHY OF JEAN-PAUL SARTRE

In a previous publication (Seinfeld 1991b) I compared Fairbairn's theory of personality development to Jean-Paul Sartre's existential phenomenology. Sartre (1943) provided powerful phenomenological support for object relations theory in his primary views that consciousness is always consciousness of an object and emotions are always emotions about an object. He described a void arising from a plenitude of being and nothingness as a lack giving rise to the desire to fill a void with an acquisition of concrete things. I (Seinfeld 1991a) compared Sartre's phenomenology to Fairbairn's view that early deprivation or the lack of primary love gives rise to the experience of emptiness based upon the biological experience of emptiness and hunger. The lack of love results in an empty core that is not a static, spatial state but rather a hunger to incorporate concrete part-objects to fill the void.

Wright (1991a) discusses how Sartre's phenomenology provided an apt description of the trauma of absence. He also contrasts the views of Winnicott and Sartre. I will discuss Winnicott at length in Chapter 6, but I will now briefly review Wright's comparison of Winnicott and Sartre because of its pertinence to my discussion of Fairbairn.

According to Wright, Winnicott was relatively warmhearted and optimistic about humanity, whereas Sartre was pessimistic and ridden with existential anxiety. Winnicott focused on the child playing while protected from impingement by the mother. For Sartre the individual is thrown into the universe with neither help nor succor, with no one to count on but himself. As Wright states, Sartre's individual is alienated, without God, the prototypical parental figure, in a universe with no meaning.

Winnicott described the actual space of separation between infant and mother as being largely avoided if the mother is good enough. Wright advances the interesting theory that consciousness may arise as a form of searching for the lost object. The baby beginning to separate becomes aware of a gap or lack. It searches for a sense of wholeness to fill the gap. For Winnicott, the gap between need and reality is bridged by the infant's creation of a transitional object. It provides the illusion of the mother's presence in her absence. There is no loss of basic trust because the mother can be felt through the transitional object and returns, in short enough intervals, so that the absence is tolerable. The area between infant and mother remains a potential space filled by the infant's transitional object, later by transitional phenomena including play, creativity, art, and religion.

As Wright points out, Winnicott's description of such a painless separation may, in part, be a moment of idealization. In fact, it resembles what Fairbairn described as an ideal state of nature when the infant separates naturally without a sense of being abandoned. Fairbairn (1941) acknowledged that a Rosseau-inspired state of nature was impossible to achieve in modern times and that the infant inevitably would be forced to separate prematurely from the caregiver. For Fairbairn, separation is an experience of painful absence that is more or less traumatic. Sartre's individual abandoned in a universe without God is comparable to Fairbairn's description of the schizoid person in modern times having lost all hope and belief in a good object. In *The Family Idiot* (1971) Sartre posited that the individual's first knowledge of nothingness or lack is in the primary relationship between infant and caregiver, in which the infant inevitably experiences some degree of a failure to be loved as a person in its own right. Thus the contrast Wright draws between Winnicott and Sartre applies identically to Winnicott and Fairbairn. It is the traumatic gap that the infant discovers between itself and the mother that gives rise to the empty core.

THE INTERNALIZATION OF OBJECT RELATIONS

Fairbairn (1941) hypothesized that the infant internalized a whole, preambivalent, but relatively unsatisfactory object to control its bad aspects. The unsatisfactory nature of the internal object gives rise to frustration and ambivalence and therefore a splitting of the object into all good and all bad. Initially, good or bad is felt as pleasurable or unpleasurable. For Fairbairn, the internal world of object relations is constituted by self and object components linked by affect (Sutherland 1963). The role played by affective experience is central. Interaction is felt as good if it is pleasurable and exciting, satisfying, or comforting. It is felt as bad if it is exciting but nongratifying, frustrating, unpleasurable, or rejecting. It is the feeling about the interaction with the external object that is internalized as an object relationship. It is such interactions linked by excitement, rejection, satisfaction, and so forth that are referred to as self and object components (Sandler and Sandler 1978). As will be shown later, Fairbairn object relations interpretations always address these internalized affective interactional units.

The infant attempts to maintain the sense of a good, pleasurable, close relationship with the external object. This provides a sense of well-being and safety. Thus the infant must attempt to abolish from the central experience other disruptive and negative interacting feeling states. Klein believed that the infant rid itself of unpleasurable states by immediately projecting them into the external object world resulting in the infantile paranoid position. Fairbairn believed that the infant endeavored to relate to the external object that it was seeking. The implication was that the infant would not project bad object experience into the outer world because it would disrupt object seeking and relating. Fairbairn argued instead that the infant split off and repressed negatively affective interactional experience. Kernberg (1980) criticized Fairbairn for telescoping repression back to the earliest stages of life and associating it with splitting. He argued that only splitting occurred in the earliest phases and that repression is a much later development.

The views of Sandler and Sandler (1978) may provide a solution to this disagreement. The authors argue, like Fairbairn, that at first the infant does not project the negative affective units into the outer world. Instead, it attempts to make them disappear internally. I propose that the infant's efforts to make the negative units disappear internally is a precursor to repression. Thus what Fairbairn described as the infant's repression and splitting of negative internalized interactions may more precisely be described as disappearing and splitting and only later becomes repression with a later form of splitting. Of course this disappearing and splitting are not entirely successful and the infant inadvertently projects bad self and object components onto the external object world.

Donald Rinsley (1981), Kernberg (1980), and I (1990a) have compared Fairbairn's internalized object relationships to Edith Jacobson's self and object representation units. I will now endeavor to be more precise in this comparison. As Sandler and Sandler (1978) point out, it is only as sensory and perceptual capacities develop that the infant forms representations of part objects. This idea is comparable to Wright's notion that the capacity for representation is the end result of symbol formation. Wright points out that unconscious symbols in the form of part-objects that are experienced as possessing the person precede the capacity for representation. Thus Fairbairn's internalized exciting, rejecting, and ideal objects are better understood as unconscious symbols that will eventually become representations. The implication for interpretation is that when the internalized object relationship is a representation, the patient is capable of beginning to look at it from the outside third position and to reflect upon it. When the internalized object relationship remains in the form of unconscious symbol, the patient can only see the other as the cause of whatever happened, or in terms of what he needs from it or what it makes him feel. Furthermore, the patient may see the external object world exclusively from the coloring of an early affective internal interaction.

I will now illustrate split-off primitive affective object relations components that are not yet representations with a clinical example.

Case Example

Diane, a patient I discussed elsewhere (1990b), reported that she needed a job. She wrote a resume but, imagining that she would appear inadequate to a prospective employer, crumpled it up and threw it away. I explored what occurred in her mind when she threw away the resume. She reported that she had imagined the boss looking at it and thinking, "Are you kidding? Does she really think I would hire her?" and throwing it away. I pointed out that these were her own thoughts about the resume and that she herself had thrown it away. Diane's anticipation of rejection colored her expectations. She imagined everyone rejecting her and could not picture anyone providing her with anything of value. Feeling that there was nothing good for her, she stayed in bed, listening to music and drinking.

During one session, Diane presented relevant historical information. She had been awarded a scholarship for postgraduate work to an Ivy League school. Her mother had hidden the letter of acceptance from her. Diane later learned of it but her mother had tried discouraging her, saying that she would not be able to do the work, that she did not belong in college, that other students and the faculty would look down on her. Diane went to school but was frightened and withdrawn, failed, and dropped out. Her life afterwards was a series of disappointments and failures.

There was a representational aspect to Diane's internal object situation. I pointed out that the image of the employer throwing away the resume represented the mother hiding the letter of acceptance. I said that she did to herself exactly what her mother had done to her—she destroyed the resume thinking the boss would do so. Therefore, the boss represented that part of her that she identified with her mother's rejecting attitude. At the same time, Diane viewed the entire world through a rejecting image: lovers, friends, the therapist. She complained that everyone treated her like shit, as if she were worthless. She then felt that others were full of shit, worthless, and rejected them in turn. Thus Diane's internal object world was symbolized in terms of feces. I pointed out that when Diane saw the world in negative depriving terms, she gave up on receiving anything positive and remained at home, depressed and drinking. The internal situation became a self-fulfilling prophecy.

AGGRESSION AND THE CLOSED
INTERNAL WORLD

Fairbairn (1944) stated that as the child develops, the central self attempts to maintain contact with the outer world and preserve a sense of well-being and safety by projecting the ideal self onto the outer world. In addition, the bad inner object relations units are split off and repressed so that they do not disrupt the outer relationship. Thus one bad inner object relations unit is of an exciting, nongratifying nature and the other is of a rejecting–rejected nature. The rejecting unit serves the central self by directing aggression against the libidinally exciting–excited unit. The libidinally excited needs that are repressed become more urgent. An antilibidinal self, identified with the rejecting parent, directs aggression against the dependent libidinal self.

Fairbairn believed that aggression was a primary drive in its own right but appeared secondary to the frustration of libidinal object-seeking needs. He rejected Freud's concept of a death instinct but believed that the clinical picture Freud based on the death instinct was common. He (1958) attributed it to an obstinate tendency on the part of individuals to keep "aggression localized within the confines of the inner world as a closed system" (p. 34). Furthermore, the aggression enclosed in this system, personified as an antilibidinal or antidependent self, was directed toward keeping libido similarly confined. The patient is trapped in a closed circuit of destruction and death that keeps out the therapist, who is viewed as an interference and intruder on the patient's bad object relationships.

In "Observations on the Nature of Hysterical States" (1954) Fairbairn provides some clinical examples of the internal bad object world. This first describes aggression localized in the closed system directed against and confining libido.

A female patient dreams of two dogs, A and B, racing. Dog A wins the race. The dreamer comforts the loser, Dog B. Dog A viciously attacks Dog B. Fairbairn states that Dog A's victory shows the antidependent self's dominance over the dependent libidinal self. The patient attempts to comfort the deprived libidinal dependent self that suffered a loss and Dog A, the antilibidinal self, cruelly attacks it. For Fairbairn, the dream illustrates the patient's dynamic psychic state. The aggressive antidependent self is constantly attacking her libidinally dependent self and not allowing it any relationship to the external object world. If the patient wants comforting from the analyst, the antidependent self will attack her just as Dog A attacked Dog B when the patient tried to comfort it. It must be emphasized that in this case the entire dynamic conflict is repressed and unconscious. The patient's central ego is oblivious that one structure sadistically attacks the other.

In Fairbairn's theory of dynamic structure, libido and aggression are inseparable from internalized object relationships. Libido and aggression may be thought of as the affective quality of object relationships or as their energic activity. Another way of saying this is that libido and aggression are always personified as self and object components (Grotstein 1981). This is what is meant by the libidinal and antilibidinal self.

THE ENDOPSYCHIC STRUCTURE

For Fairbairn, not only the libidinal and anti-libidinal self but also the exciting and rejecting objects they are respectively attached to are all repressed. Furthermore, the internal objects are very much based on their external counterparts. Fairbairn (1954) described the dream of another patient to illustrate this point.

A woman dreamed that she was trapped in a corridor between two doors. Before each door stood her father. One father held a pole before his genitals pointed at her. The other father held the same pole over his head as if threatening to hit her. Outside a window, she saw well-dressed proper couples walking with their noses in the air, as if not wanting to know of her plight. She danced in a circle, not knowing which way to turn. Fairbairn interpreted that the patient had, in reality, a father who was sexually seductive and punitive. Thus the two fathers represented a father who actually was exciting and rejecting, and she divided him into each of these qualities. She felt trapped and dominated by her need for and fear of each of these part-objects. The couples with their noses in the air represented the idealized parents. To stay in contact with them, she must deny their negative features. They are outside while she and her divided threatening father are inside representing the repressed and split-off bad object relationships and the external idealized object relationship.

THE TIE TO THE BAD OBJECT

Fairbairn (1943) believed that realistic abusive and neglectful experience accounted for the internal world of bad objects. A parent who excited the child's libidinal needs, then rejected the child, proved especially deleterious. Overstimulation resulted in excessive dependence, which made rejection all the more painful. Because of the object-seeking nature of libido, frustration was never felt purely as frustration but more importantly as emotional rejection. Fairbairn (1954) recommended that the analyst always interpret experiences of frustration in terms of rejection. A patient operating on a level of immediate need gratification in all areas of life, unable to tolerate frustration in love relationships, at work, in friendships, in all acts of daily living, attempts to deny and avoid an underlying threat of rejection. When Fairbairn spoke of an exciting, nongratifying object, he included a wide range of behaviors from emotional overinvolvement and overprotection to actual incest. When he spoke of a rejecting object, he included behaviors ranging from punitive attributes to violent abuse. Internal bad objects originally are based on the actual parental figures and are not a priori aspects of the instinctual drives. However, internal objects are not simply replicas of the real parents. Internal bad objects are split off from the good aspects of the object and are falsified, for this reason alone, because they do not possess the redeeming aspects of the real parents. Furthermore, they are doubly falsified by being distorted by the infant's own feelings, emotional tensions, and instinctual reactions. It is for these reasons that the internal bad object is often experienced as a monster or devil.

Fairbairn (1943) was struck by what he described as the libidinal tie to bad objects. He believed that the impulse was repressed because it was tied to a bad object. It was not the impulse but rather the object of the impulse that was bad. Therefore, the repression was directed toward bad objects and it was bad objects that were fundamentally repressed. Freud believed that resistance emanated from the defensive ego. The repressed id did not contribute to repression. Fairbairn argued that resistance was difficult to overcome because it emanated not only from the central ego but also from the libidinal attachment to repressed bad objects.

Fairbairn worked in a clinic during the 1940s where he saw many violently and sexually abused and delinquent youth. He was the first psychoanalyst to observe that the abused child protected, defended, and idealized the abusive parent and blamed himself for the maltreatment. Fairbairn stated that the child internalized the badness of the parent in order to idealize and protect the relationship to the real parent. At the same time, the child remained libidinally attached to the bad aspects of the parent through identification. Delinquent children often become antisocial to justify the parent's maltreatment.

I can recall hearing about a child who had been abused by his parents. When the therapist asked why he was beaten, the child concocted a story that he had been dancing on the table. It may not be long before he does in fact do something like this to justify the maltreatment. Melanie Klein believed that the depressive clings to the object to avoid the aggression and guilt associated with object loss, separation anxiety, and rage. Fairbairn (1943) believed that these concerns were secondary to the ultimate terror of being objectless and expressed this belief thus: "It was better to have a bad object than no object at all" (p. 67). He aptly described the dilemma of the abused child who found it better to feel like a sinner in a universe ruled by God than a saint in a world dominated by the Devil.

The type of patients Fairbairn described grow up and have repeated abusive relationships that recapitulate the early emotional or physical abuse. When the patient is not in an abusive relationship, he is likely to abuse himself. This shows that the abusive object is internal and projected onto suitable external objects. This type of patient may be identified with the abusive object and may maltreat, reject, excite, or frustrate others. Upon careful exploration, the therapist typically will discover that the patient mistreats himself in an identical way. Thus the therapist may interpret how the patient is overly hard on others by pointing out, at the same time, that he is equally harsh with himself. In this way the therapist begins to interpret the internal rejecting object empathically.

In doing an assessment, the therapist should always explore whether there is a pattern or history of abusive relationships. One such relationship does not necessarily mean that the patient is dominated by an internal abusive or bad object. I refer the reader to a previous publication (Seinfeld 1990c) where I describe in great detail how to interpret the internal bad object situation.

The internal bad object situation is not always enacted in external abusive relationships. The patient may internalize a parental saboteur who excites dependence and rejects autonomy. John Sutherland (1989) pointed out that psychoanalytic theory has not given enough attention to the drive for autonomy and the conflicts resulting from it. The following vignette will illustrate how the therapist interprets this conflict in object relational terms.

Case Example

Mrs. Jones was a middle-aged woman who had suffered as a child from a disabling disease. Her parents had been overprotective afterwards, telling her that she should not go out to play with other children or go to a regular school where she could be trampled, knocked down, ridiculed, or mocked, that she should avoid any after-school clubs or activities where she would be rejected. Her parents had also told her that teachers, counselors, and other adults would not understand her handicap in the same way the parents did and would not protect her properly. Mrs. Jones was disadvantaged by a limp and had difficulty walking, but subsequent medical workups revealed that she was not nearly as handicapped as she had believed. As an adult, she was emotionally crippled, agoraphobic, and afraid to work.

After several years of therapy she revealed enough historical information to become aware that her parents had been fearful of her separating long before her childhood illness and that the disease only crystallized and intensified dynamic factors already in place. Mrs. Jones made slow but gradual progress in therapy and after several years reached the point where she was ready to work as a school teacher. She came in panicked before starting the job. She said, "I'll never do it. The kids will trample me, I'll be knocked down. The principal didn't even give me a special room that would keep me from the flow of traffic. No one there cares. Who was I ever to think I could do this? I'm just kidding myself. What have I ever done? I'm a weakling emotionally and physically."

I suggested that if we transformed all of her I's into you's, we could better understand what she was going through. "You'll never do it. The kids will trample you. You'll be knocked down. The principal didn't even give you a special room that will keep you from the flow of traffic. No one there cares. Who were you to even think you could do this? You're just kidding yourself. What have you ever done? You're a weakling emotionally and physically."

In this way, I pointed out that what she said was actually an inner saboteur commanding, discouraging, frightening, and talking her out of autonomous functioning. She recognized the voice to be that of her mother, discouraging her from activities, school, friendships, all of what a child does that signifies autonomy. I noted that the terror she felt at starting the job was not only her own fear but that of her mother, the fear she had internalized from early childhood.

THE SILENT ATTACKS OF THE ANTILIBIDINAL EGO

In many cases, the antilibidinal ego is an unconscious structure sadistically repressing the libidinal ego. In such instances, the central ego's aspirations, interests, and responses may be a reaction to the silently sadistic antilibidinal ego. The following case example illustrates a repressed antilibidinal self that becomes conscious during an acid trip.

An adult male patient stated that the ideal that he aspires to is Christlike, surrendering all of his worldly possessions and sacrificing himself entirely for others. He believed this ideal may sometimes get him into trouble in that others have taken advantage of him and he felt resentful. He said that he had once been on an acid trip and had been told that he looked like Jesus Christ. However, his description of the trip revealed far more than the central ego ideal.

Several years ago he attended a rock concert immediately after tripping on acid. As he watched the concert, he began to feel the effects of the LSD. He smoked a hashish pipe and the person behind him asked if he would share it. He refused, having only a little hash left. He imagined the person as thinking, "You rich, spoiled brat." This feeling grew until he felt that everyone at the concert was thinking this. Because of the acid, he began to hallucinate, imagining that everyone spoke against him. The idea that everyone thought of him as rich and spoiled was ludicrous because he was from a working-class family. It was a hot day and people with water bottles splashed the crowd for relief. The patient believed that everyone spat on him. After the concert he felt depressed and self-destructive. Someone gave him a ride to his neighborhood and said that he looked like Jesus Christ.

I asked about the possibility of a connection between his identification with a Christlike figure and his belief during the acid trip that everyone thought he was a rich, spoiled brat. He was aware that LSD sometimes released the unconscious. I then remarked that his central conscious ideal of extreme self-sacrifice might be accompanied by an unconscious sadistic voice demanding that he surrender himself. I explained that the thoughts that became conscious during the trip and were projected onto everyone might be going on in his own mind. I said, "There might be a voice in your mind constantly telling you that you are a rich, spoiled brat. You do not consciously hear it because it is a silent, unconscious voice. You are aware that acid sometimes releases the unconscious. Even though you do not consciously hear the voice, you may unconsciously react to it by meeting its demands and completely sacrificing yourself."

The patient responded with interest that the voice referred to him as a brat. A child could be referred to as a brat. The voice was parental, but neither of his parents was cruel or sadistic. He recalled that his mother, who raised him and two siblings, had felt overwhelmed by the breakup of her marriage. Whenever he asked for spending money, toys, or presents she told him that he had to make do with what he had, that their situation was difficult. Occasionally he protested, but usually he became depressed. When he did protest his mother seemed sad and hurt. Sometimes, she scolded him, but afterwards she would be sorry and depressed. The patient experienced his anger as injurious to his mother and repressed it. He projected his anger onto his mother, thereby perceiving her as overwhelmingly angry and persecutory. He then internalized this angry object and unleashed it on his own needs. This internal antidependent structure was repressed, but its effects were felt by the central ego, which sacrificed itself to the sadistic antilibidinal demands. This case also provides an example of how the internal object may be more sadistic than its external counterpart because of the projection of rage.

PSYCHONEUROSES AS DEFENSIVE OPERATIONS

For Fairbairn (1941), the psychoneuroses—hysteria, phobias, obsessions, and paranoia—are defensive techniques against internal bad object situations that would otherwise result in depressive or schizoid conditions. In Freud and Abraham's classical viewpoint, psychopathology resulted from arrests of libidinal development of specific psychosexual fixation points: schizophrenia and schizoid conditions at the preambivalent oral phase, depressive conditions at the oral ambivalent phase, paranoia at the early anal evacuative phase, obsessions-compulsions at the late anal retentive phase, and hysteria and phobias at the phallic oedipal phase (Guntrip 1969). Fairbairn's view of psychopathology was based not on psychosexual fixation points but on relationships to bad objects.

Fairbairn (1941) described the infant's libidinal connection to the original external object as primary identification. The infant internalizes a whole but relatively unsatisfactory object. The whole unsatisfactory object is split into an ideal and bad object. The ideal object is projected onto the external world so that the infant remains in contact with the needed object world. Fairbairn suggested a process of gradual differentiation from the internal object. Infantile dependence, not the oedipal conflict, is viewed as the primary cause of psychopathology. The internalization of the object results in a state of oneness with the internal object. Fairbairn referred to this symbiosis as secondary identification. The state of primary and secondary identification is described by Fairbairn as the stage of infantile dependence, which is associated with orality. As the infant differentiates from the internal object, it enters into the transitional stage, which is similar to Mahler's separation-individuation. Throughout the transitional phase, the child experiences the conflict between dependence and autonomy. In a passage that anticipated Mahler's work, Fairbairn (1941) said,

> The great conflict of the transitional stage may now be formulated as a conflict between a progressive urge to surrender the infantile attitude of identification with the object and a regressive urge to maintain that attitude. During this period, accordingly, the behavior of the individual is characterized both by desperate endeavors on [the child's] part to separate from the object and desperate endeavors to achieve reunion with the object-desperate attempts "to escape from prison" and desperate attempts "to return home." Although one of these attitudes may come to predominate, there is in the first instance a constant oscillation between them owing to the anxiety attending each. The anxiety attending separation manifests itself as fear of isolation, and the anxiety attending identification manifests itself as a fear of being shut-in, imprisoned, engulfed. [p.43]

The psychoneuroses are techniques of this transitional phase reflecting the conflict of separating from the object. Fairbairn's theory provides a framework for interpreting psychoneurotic symptoms from the dialectic of fear of engulfment, fear of separation.

A middle-aged male patient, a successful businessman, was anxious about leaving his home while on vacation. He and his wife traveled extensively, spontaneously seeking shelter and recreation as they went along. However, the patient suffered anxiety thinking of his home, lonely and empty. He felt better hiring a house sitter. He recalled as a child that when he was in school he pictured no one at home. He feared returning to an empty house. His mother had been hospitalized for a physical illness during his first years. After she returned, she was withdrawn and reclusive. He felt that he had lost her.

The patient lived upstate and drove with his wife into Manhattan for his weekly therapy appointments. After each session, they would enjoy themselves in the city. One day his wife was unable to accompany him. He panicked as he was driving in. He attributed his anxiety to heavy traffic and difficulty finding parking. He realized that his anxiety was out of all proportion to the situation. He said, "Here I travel all over the world without fear; how do you explain that I'm panicked by driving to the city? I want you to know the extent of it. I was apprehensive all week. Then I found a parking space across the street."

I interpreted that I believed the anxiety had to do with the space of separation—traveling to and from. I remarked on the city being strange, alien. He acknowledged this but insisted he never dreaded going to strange places throughout the world. He was aware that his wife accompanied him on his world trips, that he was not entirely alone. When we pinpointed what made him anxious it was the idea that he might be late, that I would be waiting for him. It was not that I would be angry or that he valued the session much. Often he did not feel like coming. But there was something terribly unsettling about traveling so far, losing time, maybe being unable to see me and feeling lost. He said the feelings were childlike, and I interpreted that it represented the space of separation between himself and his mother, that it was too great and too traumatic as a result of her illness and subsequent unavailability. Traveling without a companion, not being able to arrive at a destination, was similar to a child wandering away and being unable to find a parent. The patient said that he felt that he was nowhere, and we agreed that nowhere was the traumatic space of separation between himself and his mother.

He then became aware of a further subtle symptom. Every day, when he arrived at his office, he felt a sense of relief. It was as if he were safely at home. He was aware that even the short daily drive to his office brought about a feeling of anxiety, as if he were nowhere until settling into his office. He said, "Here I am, a middle-aged successful businessman, inwardly feeling like a helpless, lost, abandoned child." This case illustrates Fairbairn's theory that psychoneurotic symptoms may be interpreted along the lines of the stage of transition between dependence and autonomy. For this man, his seemingly mild agoraphobic symptoms expressed his terror of differentiating from the internal object because of a fear of abandonment.

Another patient complained of being nowhere in life. He was not in a relationship with a woman, he had few friends, he did not work. He wanted to get "something going." He dreamed that he was a pilot of a rocket ship. It took off but then came to a stop in midair. It was as if he were stuck in space, not going anywhere. Next, he dreamed that he wanted to enter a house. He opened the door with a key, but there was only another door. He opened that door to find yet another. He tried again and again, only to give up. This patient feared separating, which was analogous to being lost and isolated in space. He also feared identification with the object, which was analogous to being imprisoned in a house. I interpreted that he started to separate but became afraid of being lost, that he tried to engage but was afraid to let himself enter or get truly involved. Like the previous patient, he was "nowhere," the space of traumatic separation between infant and mother.

A female adult patient was caught in what Harry Guntrip (1969) referred to as "the in and out program." She was constantly entering into and then breaking up relationships. She wished someone would call her to go out but, as soon as they did, she felt trapped, as if she might be missing something. There was a particular job she wanted. When she started to work there, she thought she wished to do something else. She again felt trapped. She also could not reside in the same house or neighborhood for long. This patient desperately longed for an identification with an object. However, as soon as the identification occurred, she felt trapped, imprisoned, and had to escape. Once she separated, she felt lost, abandoned, thereby having to return to the object. In fact, she rarely stayed in a separate position but fled from one identification to the next. The need for the identification was desperate, but so was the fear of engulfment.

There are other patients more afraid of separation than engulfment. The patient may complain of being stuck in a bad relationship, bad job, or unsatisfactory place to live. There is a component of separation in that the person always fantasizes about wanting to leave. Fairbairn found that in the phobias the conflict about separating from an internal object is projected onto an external object. When the patient wishes to merge, it is with the ideal object. When the patient wishes to flee, it is from a persecutory object. Clinicians are more apt to recognize separation conflicts around people. Fairbairn emphasized that the conflict is around an internal object, which can therefore be projected onto anything in external reality.

Fairbairn (1941) described obsessive-compulsive symptoms along the lines of conflict over differentiation. Whereas the phobic projects the internal object onto the external world, the obsessive-compulsive experiences the internal object as inner contents such as feces or urine, thoughts or feelings. As mentioned earlier, Abraham viewed expulsion of contents as sadistic destruction of the internal object. Fairbairn interpreted expulsion of contents as separation from the internal object. In the transitional stage, the conflict about differentiation from the internal object may therefore be expressed as a conflict between the urge to expel or retain contents. Whereas in orality there is a connection between incorporation and identification, in the transitional stage there is a connection between excretory expulsion and separation.

A young girl was sent away to summer camp. Her mother was depressed and suicidal, her father alcoholic. The child denied any feelings of loss or separation anxiety. She was eager to go to camp, meet other children, and engage in the camp's activities. She expressed no overt homesickness. However, shortly thereafter, she developed symptoms of nocturnal enuresis. In Fairbairn's terms, she treated the object as internal instead of external and expressed her urge to separate through urinating.

An adult male patient underwent a separation from a girlfriend who had lived with him. He felt a low-keyed depression. He endeavored to suppress feelings of loss and longing by filling his mind with things to do. These were activities at work, chores at home, shows he wished to watch on television, things he planned to buy. He even counted the stairs he climbed to his apartment. As he put it, "There was a lot of shit to do." In Fairbairn's terms, the separation from the girlfriend felt like the loss of an internal object. Thus all the things the patient held onto or counted represented the internal object he endeavored to retain. Keeping his mind filled with things to do meant that he held onto inner contents. Several months later, as he became accustomed to the separation, he was going to get rid of some things that reminded him of the relationship. He also considered giving some things away. Fairbairn's theory implies that interpretation should be made in the context of the patient's wish to separate. Obsessive-compulsive patients are often classified as withholding. Fairbairn stated that withholding is a reaction to a conflictual wish to give. Thus the patient's urge to expel implies not only loss but also a beginning inclination to give. In order to give inner contents, there must be the idea of a good containing object. Both the urge to expel and the urge to retain are associated with anxiety. Expulsion is associated with anxiety about being drained or emptied, retention with bursting or having a dread internal disease, such as cancer. The fear of being drained or emptied is equivalent to the phobic fear of being abandoned or isolated, the fear of bursting to the fear of engulfment or merger. The bulimic patient expresses a fear of being emptied when binging and a fear of bursting when vomiting. The patient may also treat other people or external things as body contents or possessions. When the object is retained, it is experienced as ideal; when evacuated, as bad.

Fairbairn described paranoia as the projection of the bad internal object onto the outer world, along with the defensive idealization of the object remaining within the patient. Thus the paranoid is grandiose but angrily distances external objects. The paranoid's projection of the bad object is a transitional effort to differentiate but not to give, as in the case of the obsessive-compulsive neurotic.

In classical analytic theory, the hysteric is described as splitting off and repressing the genitals from the whole external object. The external object is idealized and the self, which internalized the exciting bad object, is itself felt to be bad. The hysteric therefore clings to the ideal external object to escape its feelings of badness. Fairbairn contends that underlying the hysteric's conflict regarding the rejected phallus is the rejected breast.

A female patient suffered from anorexia as a child. She had an antagonistic relationship with her mother characterized by mutual hostility but got along better with her father. As a child she suffered from phobic symptoms implying difficulties around separation. She was terrified of driving under or over bridges or through tunnels. In her current adult life situation she lived with a man who met all of her needs. She could not live without him, yet she felt no romantic feelings or attraction for him. She thought of him as a good father figure. At the same time, she occasionally was attracted to men she thought of as cruel and bad. She had impulses to grab their penises and perform fellatio. She felt disgusted with herself and pushed the thought from her mind.

Fairbairn's interpretation would be that the initial anorexia reflected a rejection of the mother's breast. The fighting with her mother and the childhood phobias reflected her dependency conflicts and difficulties separating from the internal mother. She turned to the father as an idealized substitute mother, rejecting and repressing his phallus, which also contained the original maternal rejected breast. The relationship to the man she lived with represented the relationship to the idealized father. The sadistic men she occasionally desired reflected a return of the exciting, repressed phallus/breast. Their part-object status can be seen in that she referred to these men as "dicks." Fairbairn explained that the splitting off and repression of the bad exciting object permitted the central self to relate to the external world as an ideal but distant and impoverished object. The hysteric personality structure is the pathway to the schizoid position. Fairbairn based his endopsychic structural theory on the dynamics of hysteria.

The transitional stage utilizes the above psychoneuroses as defensive techniques. For most patients, the neuroses are not manifest in pure form and symptoms often overlap, given that they are different techniques for dealing with the same dependency conflict. Fairbairn believed that the transitional stage leads to the final stage of mature object relating, in which taking is followed by giving based on love or concern for the other as a separate, differentiated object.

THE UNDERLYING PSYCHOTIC CORE STATES

For Fairbairn, the psychoneuroses are defenses against the two fundamental bad object situations, that of depressive and schizoid states. The depressive reaction has to do with the patient becoming angry and enraged over feeling frustrated and rejected. There is a wish to attack the object aggressively and force it to provide love. The situation is analogous to a small child who has a temper tantrum when he cannot get what he wants from the parent (Guntrip 1969). There is the ensuing fear that hate directed against the bad object will destroy the needed good object. Fairbairn accepted Klein's theory of the depressive position and oral ambivalence and related depressive states to the failure to integrate the good and bad part-objects and resolve ambivalence. The manic reaction is not considered one of the psychoneurotic defenses but rather a direct reaction to the depressive dilemma. It will be recalled that the manic reaction was constituted by the activation of the primitive defenses.

For Fairbairn, there is an earlier, more basic dilemma. Fairbairn (1940) stated that deprivation may not give rise to hatred but to an intense craving with a need for complete possession of the object. By deprivation, Fairbairn does not mean the mother's failure to satisfy the infant's instinctual needs at the breast but rather the failure to love the infant as a person in its own right. He emphasized that being loved as an autonomous being is essential for personality growth. When the infant's need to be loved is rejected, love is made hungry. The schizoid problem is that the need to be loved has become so incorporative and urgent that love itself becomes destructive and devouring. Schizoid aloofness and the splitting of ideation and affect are the result of the fear of love destroying the object (Seinfeld 1991a). For the schizoid, the object is primarily exciting but frustrating, a desirable deserter, whereas for the depressive, the object is a denier, a robber, a rejecting object denying the depressive the good object. The psychotic depressive, more fundamentally, the schizoid condition, inevitably underlies the psychoneuroses.

THE LACK OF DEVELOPMENT OF AN INNER IDEAL OBJECT

A shortcoming of Fairbairn's theory that I discussed in a previous volume (Seinfeld 1990c) is that no description is given for the development of an internal good object in relationship to internal bad objects. In Fairbairn's earlier writings, the internal object world was constituted only by bad objects. In his later work, there is recognition that a good object is internalized to fill the void and to serve as a defense against bad objects. However, the ideal object is presented as fully formed, and there is no consideration of the problem of the development of the ideal object in the face of an inner world dominated by attacking and persecutory bad objects. Chapter 8 is devoted to this important clinical issue.

THE MATERNAL AND PATERNAL FUNCTIONS OF THE THERAPIST

Like Klein, Fairbairn acknowledged the importance of interpretation in enabling the patient to separate from the preoedipal mother. However, Fairbairn also recognized that the mother's love for the infant as an autonomous person was essential to support separation. Therefore, Fairbairn considered the object relationship between patient and therapist as the basis for effective interpretation. Fairbairn's work implies that the therapist fulfills not only a paternal function of separating the child from the preoedipal mother through interpretation of resistance but also a maternal function of supporting the patient so that he need not feel utterly abandoned or isolated as he enters the space of separateness. Fairbairn never explicated the specifics of the holding or good object relationship, instead leaving this task to other clinicians. It is those clinicians who experimented with the maternal, holding function that we will now discuss.

PART TWO

HOLDING

5

SANDOR FERENCZI AND MICHAEL BALINT: THE MATERNAL FUNCTION

Sandor Ferenczi was the first analyst to recognize and experiment with the maternal or holding function of the psychotherapist. He protested against the idea of the untreatable patient and believed that any patient who asked for help should receive it, regardless of the severity of pathology. He asserted that if a patient was untreatable, it was because the analyst or analysis had not yet devised the necessary knowledge or effective means of intervention. In other words, it was psychoanalysis, not the patient, that was inadequate. Ferenczi became well known in the psychoanalytic community for being the analyst of last resort for seemingly hopeless cases. In working with cases considered untreatable by classical technique, Ferenczi engaged in original but unorthodox experiments and developed a reputation as the *enfant terrible* of psychoanalysis (Stanton 1991).

Ferenczi originally questioned classical psychoanalytic technique because of his work with a special patient population—traumatized soldiers in World War I. As director of a special war neurosis clinic in Budapest, he became aware that trauma produced splitting, which resulted in the patient's being overwhelmed by infantile and unconscious material. Given that long-term analytic treatment was often inappropriate, Ferenczi said that the patients needed active tenderness so that a therapist could enable them to relax and reach split-off parts of the self. It is interesting that during World War II, Fairbairn was responsible for appraising the psychological states of traumatized soldiers. Fairbairn also discovered that the patients suffered from splitting and attributed the susceptibility to war neurosis to the trauma of being separated from significant objects that reawakened unsatisfactory early life experiences.

Following the war, at the First International Psychoanalytic Association Congress held in Budapest in September 1918, Ferenczi (1920) proposed the active technique of psychoanalysis. This method, although influenced by his work on war neurosis, was not based on the provision of tenderness but rather on prohibition. Ferenczi pointed out that some patients abuse the free association rule by endeavoring to extend psychoanalysis indefinitely. He (Ferenczi 1920) suggested that with these cases, the analyst no longer hold to the fundamental rule of free association but instead direct the course of analysis. The analyst could do so by imposing tasks. For instance, the analyst might require the patient to complete sentences if he is resisting to do so, or set a termination date if the patient is resisting free association. The analyst might prohibit the patient from employing masturbatory substitutes during the session. For instance, the analyst might institute prohibitions against tongue chewing, nail biting, or head scratching. The analyst could even extend the prohibition to behavior outside the therapeutic situation, for instance, by forbidding sexual intercourse. This technique sought to help the patient bring to consciousness preverbal experience that was not accessible through free association. Thus Ferenczi was among the first analysts to begin the exploration of the earliest phases of development beyond verbal language.

Ferenczi's experience with traumatized soldiers extended to an interest in the traumatic experiences of children at the hands of adults. His clinical experience led him to believe that child abuse, especially sexual abuse, was more common than analysts recognized. In "Confusion of Tongues between Adults and the Child" (1933) he wrote,

> I obtained above all new corroborative evidence for my supposition that the trauma, especially the sexual trauma, as the patho-

genic factor cannot be valued highly enough. Even children of very respectable, sincerely puritanical families fall victim to real violence or rape much more often than one had dared to suppose. Either it is the parents who try to find a substitute gratification . . . for their frustration, or it is people felt to be trustworthy . . . who misuse the ignorance or innocence of the child. The immediate explanation that these are only sexual fantasies of the child . . . is unfortunately made invalid by the number of such confessions. [p. 161]

Ferenczi (1933) drew parallels between the child traumatized by the hypocrisy of adults, the soldier traumatized by the hypocrisy of war, and the mentally ill person traumatized by the hypocrisy of society. He described a process that occurred with patients who had been traumatically abused that was to influence his own treatment experiments. The traumatized person suffered a breakdown of defenses, resulting eventually in a surrendering of the patient to the situation and a state of depersonalization in which he withdrew outside himself to view the situation from a detached perspective. From this distance, the patient may be able to view the abuser as sick or mad and sometimes even try to cure the abuser. Ferenczi noted that abused children tend to become therapists to their parents and are often strikingly altruistic. He believed that a patient could suffer a similar trauma at the hands of a too distant or rigid analyst. When theory is translated into a dogmatic technique, or the analyst denies his own countertransference, or the patient is designated untreatable, the analyst inflicts a trauma on the patient that revives the traumas of the past. Ferenczi's use of the active technique emphasizing prohibition gradually gave way to a supportive relaxation technique.

THE RELAXATION TECHNIQUE

As Stanton (1991) points out, Ferenczi's relaxation technique involved nurturing and calming efforts as opposed to the prohibitions of the earlier active technique. This technique was especially appropriate for patients who had suffered from traumatic abuse. Ferenczi believed that a child's psyche was whole but that the traumas inherent throughout development never left an adult mind undivided. He emphasized the need for the therapist to provide friendly encouragement and relaxation to reach the split-off selves. Only with the active support of the therapist could the adult patient feel safe enough to risk the remembrance and reliving of early traumatic abuse. Ferenczi believed that the paternal function of the therapist's interpretive efforts may not always be expressed in a language the patient understands. He (1933) stated, "The patient who goes off in a trance is a *child indeed* who no longer reacts to intellectual explanations, only perhaps to maternal friendliness; without it he feels lonely and abandoned in his greatest need" (p. 160). Ferenczi questioned Freud's belief that severely disturbed patients did not develop a positive transference. He argued that with such patients, the analyst must first experience a positive countertransference to elicit the patient's positive transference. A severe repression of the analyst's countertransference might inhibit the emergence of the transference. Ferenczi emphasized that a severely disturbed patient was unusually astute in recognizing the unconscious negative countertransference. The patient may not directly acknowledge or express protest about the analyst's unconscious negative reactions but instead may withdraw. Ferenczi believed it was essential for the analyst to help the patient verbalize his protest if there are indications that the patient detects hypocrisy on the part of the analyst.

THE LANGUAGE OF TENDERNESS

Ferenczi's supportive relaxation technique was informed by his theoretical views, which anticipated contemporary object relations theory. He (1929) described tenderness as the preoedipal register of experience constituted by oral gratification, kissing, cuddling, and tactile closeness. These feelings expressed infantile sexuality but did not become urgent, greedy, or desperate unless they were excited by overindulgent or abusive behavior on the part of the adult. He emphasized that a large part of the child's sexuality was not spontaneous, but was complicated or grafted on by the overstimulating behavior of adults. Ferenczi termed this adult–overstimulated sexuality "passion," that is, the oedipal and postoedipal register of phallic or genital experience. Ferenczi argued that, for many patients, especially those who were sexually abused, there is a confusion between two registers of experience. The child experiences a desire for tenderness, but the adult may respond passionately. Thus the language of passion is grafted onto the language of tenderness. The parent may provoke the language of passion by being over-stimulating, overly frustrating, or a combination of the two.

Ferenczi's views are quite compatible with current object relations theory. The language of tenderness suggests that libido is object seeking. The notion that the abusive parent excites the child's urgent sexuality with the language of passion is similar to the concept of the exciting object. Ferenczi's notion that overly frustrating behavior on the part of the adult is also a pathogenic factor suggests the rejecting object. Object relations theory emphasizes that the child's language of passion or guilt is indicative of the child's having internalized the parental reactions. Ferenczi stated that the abusive parent often denies guilt about abusing the child but that the child is attuned to the unconscious guilt of the parent and identifies with it out of loyalty to the parent. The therapeutic aim is to enable the patient to separate from the identification with the parent's guilt.

THE TECHNIQUE OF MUTUAL ANALYSIS

As Stanton (1991) points out, Ferenczi's model of analysis is anarchic. Its philosophical influence was not terrorism or violence but rather Kropotkin's advocacy of pacifistic mutual aid. Ferenczi believed in revolutionizing psychoanalysis, which he hoped could someday revolutionize society. Psychoanalysis was an arena in which mutual aid could begin to be practiced. Ferenczi was concerned that the relaxation technique resembled hypnosis and felt that as the patient lapsed into a hypnoticlike, submissive state, the analyst still remained the objective, knowledgeable observer. His feeling that there was still too much potential authority in the relaxation technique contributed to the development of "mutual analysis," a technique that rejected the authoritative adult position of the therapist and recommended that the therapist engage in a mutual regressive experience in the transference–countertransference situation.

A CLINICAL EXPERIMENT

Fortunately, Ferenczi kept a diary dated from January to October 1932, shortly before his death, that recorded his clinical experiments. In one entry, dated May 5, he described how the idea of mutual analysis was conceived.

The patient, Elizabeth Severn (referred to as R.N. in the diary), had been in analysis with Ferenczi for over two years. She was American, had a doctorate in philosophy, and had written academic books on psychology and psychoanalysis. Ferenczi reported that the patient was initially disagreeable and made little progress. He redoubled his efforts to help, maybe counterphobically, determined that he would not be discouraged by any difficulty. He gradually gave in to all of her wishes, doubling the number of sessions, going to her house instead of insisting that she come to him, taking her with him for vacation trips, and seeing her on Sundays. With such formidable efforts on Ferenczi's part, the traumatic infantile history eventually emerged. The patient relived traumatic experiences of being drugged and sexually abused by her father at the age of 18 months and then raped by him at age 5. Following the abusive experience, the patient's organizing drive centers on developing an extremely assertive and rigorously routinized lifestyle characterized by excessive independence and self-assurance and "immensely strong will power as reflected by the marble-like rigidity of her facial features . . . [and] all together a somewhat sovereign, majestic superiority of a queen or even the royal imperviousness of a king" (p. 197). In object relations terms, her central ego was dominated and pervaded by an unusually strong antilibidinal ego. Ferenczi provided supportive technique with the idea of reaching the language of tenderness.

The patient concluded that Ferenczi was in love with her, since he had given in to all of her needs, and that she found in him the ideal lover. Ferenczi became frightened and retreated, attempting to interpret the negative emotions she ought to have felt for him. She responded with identical interpretations, as if she were the analyst and he the patient. Ferenczi decided that her interpretations were justified. He subsequently gave freer expression to his emotions and felt that the analysis, which had been stagnant for two years, was now progressing. He began to conduct the experiment in a more systematic fashion, and he and the patient took turns analyzing each other.

Ferenczi stated that during the mutual analytic sessions, the patient's overly aggressive imperious attitude was modified. He said that in Elizabeth Severn he found his mother again. His actual mother had been hard and rejecting, and he had feared her. The patient knew this and at times treated him very gently. He said the analysis enabled her to transform her own hardness into a friendlier softness.

In her introduction to Ferenczi's diary, Judith Dupont (1991) says that on no account can Ferenczi be accused of embarking upon the experiment of mutual analysis out of preference for an easy path. Ferenczi sometimes put himself in the hands of a difficult, severely disturbed patient who would have been considered untreatable by most analysts of the period. Gradually, he fell upon a whole series of problems in the technique of mutual analysis. He stated that the patient deflected attention from herself by focusing on him, that the search for complexes in the analyst became nearly paranoid, that the patient developed delusions about their collaboration and attempted to prolong the analysis indefinitely. Ferenczi decided to stop the experiment of mutual analysis. After a period of hostility and disorganization, the patient decided to carry on the analysis and made significant progress. In an entry dated June 3, Ferenczi concluded that mutual analysis was only made necessary by the insufficiently thorough analysis of the analyst. He determined that the treatment by an analyst who remained neutral was preferable.

Ferenczi's experiments remain important for contemporary therapeutic technique. He was among the first to recognize the significance of countertransference. He cautioned that the analyst's over- or underactivity could affect the nature of the transference. He viewed the patient–therapist relationship as intersubjective, in the sense that the transference and countertransference constantly interacted with each other.

These experiments prompted a debate with Freud concerning the value of the maternal versus paternal functions of the psycho-therapist. They exchanged a series of letters that illuminate their debate. Ferenczi described his therapeutic work with clients, while Freud ignored his idea and instead reiterated his lack of interest in the therapeutic aspects of analysis. On January 17, 1930, Ferenczi wrote to Freud concerning their relationship. He said that Freud had been revered, if ambivalently loved, as mentor, model, and analyst. Due to unfavorable circumstances, however, the analysis could not be completed. He complained that Freud ignored his negative transference and never helped him to discuss it. Despite this, he managed to accept the fact that he was not more important to Freud. Incidents were mentioned in which Ferenczi found Freud to be overly strict and authoritarian. He wondered whether it would have been better if Freud had been more mild and indulgent. Letters were then exchanged between them in a cordial, friendly tone. In a letter dated September 15, 1931, Ferenczi described in considerable detail the work recorded in his diary. On September 18 Freud replied with a sense of disillusionment, cautioning that Ferenczi was charting an unwise course but believing that he even-tually would correct his ways. Subsequent letters reflected a further exacerbation of the disagreement between them, culminating in Freud's criticism of Ferenczi for what he described as the "kissing technique." Dupont (1991) points out that Freud's reference to the kissing technique may have been the result of a misunderstanding by Freud upon hearing from a patient (Claire Thompson, who later became a well-known analyst) that "Papa Ferenczi" had allowed her to kiss him.

Commentary

Although there may have been a misunderstanding, there were nevertheless clear differences in their views. Freud was skeptical about Ferenczi's basic premise that an analyst could provide the patient with a maternal substitute experience that could remedy early deprivation or trauma. A close reading of Freud's case studies—the Ratman and the Wolfman—suggests that he was not averse to assuming a humanistic and nurturing attitude toward patients. Ferenczi's work goes farther by beginning to recognize the value of holding to address preoedipal issues. At the same time, Ferenczi did not distinguish adequately between the therapist's assuming a symbol position in performing a maternal function to foster psychic structure and the therapist's attempting to actually be the mother and attempt to meet early frustrated needs. Freud's criticism was therefore understandable because he recognized that Ferenczi's techniques could result in destructive regression.

Ferenczi was remarkably intuitive. As Stanton (1991) points out, people who had direct experience with Ferenczi described him as an "unequalled virtuoso" (p. 152). His method of therapy was charting dangerous and uncertain territory. It will be recalled that Fairbairn felt that the development of theory should precede practice and that technique addressing early deficits should be developed gradually and prudently. It is likely that Freud's genius was in the area of theory building, whereas Ferenczi's was in the area of practice. As Wright notes (1991d), it is often necessary for the therapist to help the patient tolerate the psychic space of separateness so that the patient can later play within this potential space and holding environment. Although Ferenczi's views anticipated object relations theory, psychoanalytic knowledge had not yet reached back to the earliest phases of personality formation to provide greater clarity as to how the therapist could provide a holding function while minimizing the dangers of regression. Wright (1991b) explains that during the process of symbol formation, the space between infant and mother is filled by a transitional object that has the feel of the mother herself. The therapist performing the holding function tries to provide the feel of mothering while maintaining for the patient the distinction that the therapist is not the actual parent.

MICHAEL BALINT

Michael Balint was a student of Ferenczi in Budapest and witnessed his experiments firsthand. He reported that, in the last years of his analytic work, Ferenczi allowed each patient to have as much time as needed, several sessions daily, if necessary, at night and on weekends. Balint felt that the experiments were inconclusive in that Ferenczi had to give up his analytic work a few weeks before his death.

Balint (1968) continued to experiment with therapeutic regression in the tradition of Ferenczi after he emigrated from Budapest to England, where he became a leading figure in the object relations independent tradition. He found that certain patients regress in a two-person relationship to a primitive level of ego development, which he referred to as the basic fault. The infant is in need of primary love from the caregiver for the survival of the ego in the same way that the organism requires oxygen for biological survival. Primary love is provided through mirroring, attunement, and holding. There can be a failure in primary love either because of congenital failures impeding the infant's capacity to extract from the environment or because of insufficient support or nurturing on the part of the environment. The failure of primary love gives rise to the basic fault, which refers to an irregularity or defect in overall psychic structure. The basic fault is experienced by the infant as a state of emptiness, lack, or deadness, and is manifested in oral greed or addictive states.

Based on his clinical work with patients, Balint (1968) distinguished two forms of regression that occur in the therapeutic situation. In the therapeutic form, the patient regressed for one or more periods. But from this regression the patient emerged much improved. Balint described this phenomenon as benign regression. In the second form, the patient never has enough of his own needs met. As soon as a need or wish is satisfied, it is replaced by a new wish or craving, equally urgent. The regression in such cases resulted in an addictive state that was difficult to handle and often proved, as predicted by Freud, intractable. Balint mentioned the case of Anna O., treated by Joseph Breuer, as an example of malignant regression. Chapter 10 examines this case.

Balint assumed that in cases of malignant regression, there was a serious difference between the strength of the instincts and the strength of the ego. Balint followed this clue to remark upon the intensity of the patient's demands, which Freud characterized as "craving." The form of the wish was pregenital, but the high intensity of the wish suggested to Balint a genital-orgastic nature. Drawing on the case of Anna O. as prototypical, Ferenczi found that such cases are classical hysteric patients who expressed genital-libidinal strivings through seemingly preoedipal wishes. They primarily seek the gratification of instinctual cravings from the object. Ferenczi distinguished them from those who seek not instinctual gratification, but rather recognition from the object.

THERAPEUTIC AND MALIGNANT REGRESSION

Balint's views on the development of object relations informed his discussion on benign and malignant regression in the transference. It is essential to be aware of how many persons the patient is related to within his imagination and the number of persons he could relate to in external reality. The infant who is unable to distinguish self and object works in a one-person frame. Later, when the infant can relate to the mother as a separate object but cannot tolerate a third object, he exists in a two-person frame. It is only when the child is in the oedipal frame that three-person relations are established (Rayner 1991).

Balint believed that the classical interpretive approach was effective for patients in the oedipal realm. Their use of language is on a symbolic level and there is agreement as to what words mean. There are some patients who do not understand the analyst's language as he intends and instead hear his interpretations as expressions of love, hate, or indifference. Ferenczi (1933) described this phenomenon as "a confusion of tongues," (p. 156). Balint perceived the analytic treatment as leading in one of two directions: either enabling thoughts to find verbal expression or regressing to earlier levels in the transference to find a new and better solution. It is the patients who do not respond to words on a symbolic level that need to regress to the level of the basic fault. Balint stated that in the treatment of the neurotic oedipal patient, the analyst is barely pressured out of a neutral position. Attunement can be taken for granted. In work involving the basic fault, it is much more difficult for the analyst to maintain neutrality and remain attuned to the patient. The provision of primary love is the essential therapeutic ingredient.

For Balint, primary love occurs in utero and afterwards becomes the need to be loved without conflict. Like Fairbairn, Balint speaks of a preambivalent need on the part of the infant to be loved, which, to a degree, continues the security in utero. Balint's meaning is also close to Ferenczi's primary passive love, but he dropped the term "passive" as he became increasingly impressed by the infant's active object seeking. In optimal circumstances, according to Balint (1968) the infant and mother remain relatively undifferentiated in a "harmonious mix-up" (p. 56).

In therapeutic regression, the patient must be allowed to regress to a state of harmonious mix-up, or primary love, with the analyst. Words become relatively meaningless at this level, as the patient is acutely sensitive to the analyst's nonverbal responses. Balint pointed out that oedipal or preoedipal interpretations could fail the patient. In this, he differed from the Kleinians. As Rayner (1991) notes, the interpreting analyst can be a master of word play but can sometimes overwhelm the patient, who then becomes the weak or dependent partner in the analytic situation. If the patient protests, the resistance is interpreted and fault is sometimes found with the patient instead of with the analytic relationship. Balint believed that the only way forward for the patient may be progression through regression.

Balint remained cautious in recommending the therapeutic aspects of regression, emphasizing that it should always be thought of as a temporary measure. In the worst of circumstances, regression provokes greed and dependency that can feed off the analyst's support. In the best of circumstances, it offers new ways of object relating and new ways of being and doing and new ways of loving and hating. The aim of therapeutic regression is a return to the point before faulty development occurred that provides an opportunity for psychic rebirth. In therapeutic regression, the patient seeks recognition. Hegel and Kojève introduced the need for recognition to confirm the self in philosophy. Balint in turn introduced the need for recognition in the therapeutic setting, and Winnicott explored its origins in the infant–mother relationship. Balint found that patients suffering from severe hysterical neurosis manifest genital dynamic needs in the transference. The therapist may be misled because these patients express oedipal–genital needs in preoedipal form. He cautioned the therapist that for these patients regression can be malignant.

Balint argued that in malignant regression the patient seeks instinctual gratification, not recognition. The mood of harmonious mix-up breaks down and urgent clinging follows. Destructive regression is characterized by insatiable demands for gratification.

Critique

Balint is basing his distinction between benign and malignant regression on whether the patient is schizoid or hysterically neurotic and on the level of the basic fault. He is also drawing on Fairbairn's distinction between object and satisfaction seeking. The schizoid patient at the level of the basic fault is perceived as object seeking, while the hysterical neurotic patient is seen as satisfaction seeking. It will be recalled that Fairbairn viewed the neurosis as a defensive technique against an underlying psychotic state. Furthermore, he viewed the hysterical condition as the prototype of the schizoid endopsychic structure. The schizoid condition was often found to be underlying hysteria. For Fairbairn, the hysteric and schizoid patient would not be two altogether different types of patients. In fact, what Balint describes as malignant regression would fit Fairbairn's description of the libidinal ego attached to the exciting object. This object relations configuration is one of insatiable need defended against by the antilibidinal ego. What Balint describes as malignant regression would be understood by Fairbairn as the emergence of the libidinal ego-exciting object transference. Balint was correct in thinking that it would be ineffective to gratify this type of regression. Fairbairn's views also imply that underlying the patient's hysterical oedipal needs is the preoedipal longing for the breast. These theoretical considerations suggest that malignant transferences should first be met by interpretation and not gratification but that once they lose their intensity and hold on him, the patient may be able to enter into the harmonious mix-up of therapeutic regression. (I devote Chapter 11 to the treatment of the hysterical–oedipal patient.) It will be recalled that satisfaction seeking originally serves object seeking until they are split off through deleterious object relations experience. It is therefore misleading to differentiate patients as satisfaction seeking or object seeking without taking into account splitting. Through the interpretation of splitting, the therapist may be able to help the patient make optimal use of the therapeutic relationship.

A CLINICAL EXPERIMENT IN THERAPEUTIC REGRESSION

Balint provided clinical examples of therapeutic regression. In the latter part of the 1920s he started analytic treatment with a young woman described as attractive and vivacious. She complained of an inability to achieve anything. She completed a university course for a degree but could not take the final examination. She was popular with men but was unable to respond. It became apparent that her inability to achieve and to respond rested on an unwillingness to take any risk or make any decision. The patient had a close relationship with her obsessive-compulsive father, while her relationship to her unreliable mother remained ambivalent. She compensated for this insecure upbringing in her rigid efforts to hold onto the status quo.

After about two years of treatment Balint remarked that the important thing for the patient was to keep both feet planted firmly on the ground and her head safely up. She responded that since her earliest childhood, she had never been able to do a somersault, though she desperately longed to. Balint suggested she try it on the spot. She rose from the couch and did so, achieving a perfect somersault to her amazement. Balint reported that following this incident the patient made significant strides in her social, emotional, and professional life.

Freud insisted that the patient not act but instead put all of her feelings into words. Balint (1968) defied the paternal function by permitting the patient to act out her wish. He remarked that the term *regression* was not entirely accurate in this case because the patient did not repeat an old pattern of behavior but instead did something for the first time. Regression also refers to a primitive mode of experience after more mature modes have been established. Balint (1968) pointed out that here the patient's action can be described in terms of a "removal of repression which, because of its symbolic function had become inhibited, ego dystonic, was now liberated and after detaching its secondary erotic cathexis was integrated into the ego as something enjoyable" (p. 31). However, Balint believed that this economic explanation, although valid, was secondary to the fact that the breakthrough occurred in the psycho-analytic relationship and therefore provided opportunity for new ways of loving and hating.

Balint's technique of therapeutic regression involved facilitating the regressive act that grew out of the patient's material. In the clinical example given here, Balint did not come up with a task for the patient. Instead, it was the patient who recalled never doing a somersault but always wishing to and it was Balint who recommended that the patient try it. If Balint had concocted the idea of the somersault, I suspect that such an intervention would have put the analyst in an omniscient, powerful position and would have fostered destructive regression. As Rayner (1991) explains, Balint saw the signs of readiness in the patient for benign regression but was careful to avoid malignant regression. He thereby advanced the understanding of regression beyond Ferenczi's pioneering efforts. Among analysts who allowed for therapeutic regression, Balint was the most cautious, probably because of his firsthand knowledge of Ferenczi's difficult experiments.

6

DONALD WINNICOTT AND THE HOLDING RELATIONSHIP

Among psychoanalysts, Donald Winnicott is the most important representative of the maternal function of the psychotherapist. A pediatrician and psychoanalyst, Winnicott grew up in a large extended family in Plymouth, Devon. It is likely that the joyous and growth-promoting contact with his lively family impressed upon him the importance of object relations. It may also have influenced him in his development of the concept of holding.

DEVELOPMENTAL THEORY

Winnicott (1962) described the infant as unintegrated for a good part of the time. The mother holds the infant, providing a sense of wholeness to his sensory motor parts. Thus holding implies a holding together to prevent coming apart. Primary maternal preoccupation occurs toward the end of pregnancy through several weeks of postpartum. The mother experiences a heightened sense of awareness about herself and the baby. In the context of the mother's holding, there is a spontaneous gesture on the part of the infant that the mother meets. The infant reaches out for the breast or the object, and it is there to be found. Therefore, the infant experiences itself as creating the breast or the object. The spontaneous gesture gives rise to a sense of omnipotence, which is an important precursor to creativity. Winnicott distinguished between the mother who responds to the infant's gesture—the environmental mother—and the mother who is the object of the infant's instinctual drives—the part-object mother. The infant's relationship to the subjective object is essential to its sense of aliveness and reality. Winnicott (1971b) used the term *object relating* for the infant's sense of omnipotent oneness with the mother. Winnicott's object relating is comparable to Fairbairn's primary identification and Mahler's symbiosis.

It is inevitable that the mother will eventually fail the infant and the infant will come to see her as a separate other. It is the infant's aggressive attacks on the mother that result in the mother becoming a separate, objectively perceived object outside the infant's omnipotent control. The mother is now perceived as external and can be used as a separate object. The infant thus advances from object relating to object usage. Winnicott (1971b) poetically described how the infant must destroy the mother to place her outside its omnipotent projections and thereby establish a sense of externality that hinges upon the actual mother serving the infant's attacks.

WINNICOTT AND SARTRE

Wright (1991a) finds that the infant's transition from object relating to object usage is associated with a separation or gap between infant and mother. He hypothesizes that this rudimentary separation becomes the space of consciousness itself. The baby searches for the mother, her face, or her breast. In a previous publication I (Seinfeld 1991b) compared object relations views about separation from the object to Sartre's phenomenological ideas about lack and nothingness. Wright (1991a) also compares Winnicott and Sartre, suggesting that Sartre's phenomenology provided an apt description of the trauma of absence.

For Winnicott, it is not inevitable that the infant will experience separation as traumatic abandonment. The baby originally experiences separation as a gap or lack, according to Wright.

The infant searches for the mother. If all goes well, the infant finds something that has the feel of the mother. A sensory pattern may be found in a soft toy or a cuddly blanket that has the feel of the mother. Wright says that the baby uses the sensory pattern of the transitional object to fill the space that was left by the absent object. The potential space eventually may become an actual space, a painful lack the baby must tolerate, which is filled by an image or representation of the mother that in turn results in the full development of symbolization. The self realizes the distinction between the symbol and what is symbolized.

The infant's creation of a transitional object provides the illusion of the mother's presence in her absence and eases separation anxiety. As long as the mother returns within a reasonable period, separation is tolerable and there is no traumatic loss of basic trust. The non-traumatic space of separation between infant and mother is a potential space filled by the infant's transitional object and later by transitional phenomena including play, creativity, art, and religion.

Although Winnicott described the child's development from a relatively optimistic outlook, he certainly did not deny the impact of environmental trauma and its adverse effects on personality development. It is inevitable that the mother will sometimes fail the child. In fact, failures to meet the child's instinctual needs served adaptation and frustration tolerance and introduced the child to the reality principle: What person could ever be induced to separate from a perfect object? Winnicott stressed that the effects of such failure were malignantly compounded if the parent did not empathize with the injured child. It is essential that there be an opportunity for repair. In other words, after such failure, it is imperative for the mother to permit regression to a state of merger or dependence. When failures are repaired in this way they become benign and enhance reality testing.

Winnicott compared the mother's failing of the infant to the inevitable situation of the therapist failing the patient. He said it was essential that the therapist also provide opportunity for repair and merger. I will illustrate the therapist's holding function with a clinical vignette.

Case Examples

The patient, a middle-aged male adult, was canceling and rescheduling appointments every week. The therapist was unsure about the time of the next scheduled appointment and called the patient to be sure there would be no mixup. The patient came in for the next session enraged. He complained that the therapist was not paying attention to scheduling. The therapist felt annoyed and defensive and wished to say, "Well, you were canceling appointments repeatedly, so I forgot. You were acting as if our sessions were not important, so I began to feel that way." This remark would blame and ridicule the patient. The therapist should remark on the interaction but not blame the patient. The therapist might say, "There have been many changes of appointments, and I also forgot the appointment time. You then felt that I did not care enough to remember your time, that I did not hold you or your time in mind, that it was out of sight, out of mind."

The therapist should not say that the patient is to blame or that the changes of appointments directly caused the therapist to forget. This remark would be saying that the therapist was not responsible himself for forgetting. I am viewing the repeated changing of appointments as a conditioning factor or context of the therapist's forgetting, but not as a mechanistic sole determinant.

The patient had experienced extreme parental neglect. During his adolescence, he sometimes left home for several days. His parents did not know his whereabouts nor did they attempt to find out. The transference–countertransference situation was a reliving of the climate of early parental neglect. Knowing this, the therapist should not say that the patient is inducing in him the early neglect of the parent. The therapist also should not say that both patient and therapist are reliving the neglect in the patient's early history. These remarks will only confirm the patient's deep-seated fear that the therapist is as unreliable as the original parent and that the situation is hopeless. The therapist instead might remark, "My forgetting your appointment was injurious in its own right. It could be that it becomes complicated and even more hurtful because it reminds you of the experience of your parents' forgetting you when you were a helpless, vulnerable child. I believed you would be angry on the basis of my forgetting your appointment, but that anger turns to rage because it gets mixed up with what was done to you in your childhood. It is very important that I pay attention to these comings and goings in the future so that you are not made to feel the same way you did during childhood."

This remark avoids confirming the patient's idea that the therapist is identical to the original parent. Ferenczi was aware that the therapist could inadvertently repeat the early trauma the patient had experienced. However, he did not take into account that his remedy of mutual analysis could inflict further trauma in that the severely disturbed patient has little capacity to distinguish the therapist from the actual parent and will be prone to viewing the therapist as the parent. Winnicott's technique enables the patient to begin to distinguish the therapist from the parent by demonstrating understanding for how the patient was made to feel, first by the parent and later by the therapist.

In the same way that the therapist empathizes with the patient over failures on his part, he also provides empathy for failing to gratify the patient. As Wright (1991d) points out, in his paternal function the therapist discourages action, especially in the area of instinctual gratification. However, the therapist must help the patient tolerate frustration by providing empathy for how the patient feels.

A patient had been in therapy for several years when she became aware of the maltreatment she had experienced at the hands of her parents. As she remembered the abuse she had endured, she became extremely upset at the end of each session. She hated the therapist for dredging up the painful feelings and leaving her alone to cope.

Wright (1991) notes that once the patient becomes aware of unmet needs she directs them toward the therapist with the hope of having them finally fulfilled. The therapist meets such needs not by offering gratification but by interpreting the reliving of early deprivation and frustration. This is a crucial moment in therapy: the patient may leave, experiencing the therapist as another exciting but frustrating object, or stay and finally work through the tie to early bad objects.

At this point, the therapist tried to hold the patient by saying, "You are not accustomed to anyone valuing and holding onto what you leave behind."

She replied, "It is as if I pour out my heart, tell you all about the abuse, but when I leave all is forgotten and I am lost and left alone with the painful feelings."

The therapist said, "Your feeling that it is out of sight, out of mind suggests that throughout your life you have never had the experience of anyone caring enough to remember you. You are therefore unable to hold onto a positive sense of our work together or a belief that what you say is important enough for me to remember."

She remarked that she would feel less abandoned and alone if she believed the therapist remembered.

The therapist did not directly gratify the patient by reassuring her that he cared and would remember all that she said. Instead, he remarked upon her deficit in being capable of believing the other will remember because the real objects of her early life had failed to remember.

THE TRUE SELF AND MIRRORING

Winnicott (1960) considered the true self to be derived from the aliveness and vitality of body tissues and their functioning. For Winnicott (1971c), being is not merely existing but rather feeling real, authentic, and alive. It is this feeling of aliveness and spontaneity that constitutes the true self. Mirroring confirms being and provides a sense of feeling real and alive. The patient lacking this vitality feels unreal, unauthentic, and only goes through the motions of living. Winnicott stated that doing must rest on a secure sense of being. Interpretation promoting autonomy when being remains unauthentic results in a false–self organization. It was this radical discovery that led Winnicott beyond the paternal function to explore the beginning formation of the ego in the infant–mother relationship and to provide holding aimed at establishing authentic being so that separation would be authentic.

Like Balint, Winnicott believed that frustration of ego needs is more harmful than the frustration of id needs. There is a need for recognition separate from the need for instinctual gratification. Jean-Paul Sartre said that the self originates and develops under the gaze of the other. By gaze he did not mean vision but rather the object's total response. Winnicott (1971c) expressed this idea in a developmental perspective, saying that recognition manifests itself in the mother's mirroring of the true self, thereby confirming the infant's sense of aliveness. It is the recognition or mirroring by the other that allows the self to turn inward, to reach, and to recognize itself. A brief dialogue between Cassius and Brutus from Shakespeare's *Julius Caesar* illustrates the need for mirroring:

> *Cassius*: Tell me, good Brutus, can you see your face?
> *Brutus*: No, Cassius, for the eye sees not itself. But by reflection, by some other things.

Cassius is endeavoring to convince Brutus that the plan to assassinate Caesar is warranted, since Brutus is by nature a good man and therefore would only think of doing what is good or just. But Brutus replies that his good nature exists in the reflection of the mirroring other, that he needs the response of the other to know who he is.

In his important paper, "Mirror Role of Mother and Family" Winnicott (1971) said, "What does the infant see when he or she looks into the mother's face? I am suggesting that ordinarily, what the infant sees is himself or herself. In other words, the mother is looking at the baby and what she looks like is related to what she sees there" (p. 172).

Winnicott argued that when the infant seeks mirroring, it is essential that he discover, reflected in the mother's look, his own true nature and not her troubled mood, whom she perceives him to be instead of who he is, or worst of all, no sign of him. Winnicott stated that the infant experiences a sense of going-on-being in the mirroring and protective presence of the mother. If the child is imposed upon, he suffers traumatic impingement, which adversely affects the ego, giving rise to a sense of disintegration, of falling to pieces and fragmentation. One might think of the nursery rhyme in which Humpty Dumpty had a great fall and "all the King's horses and all the King's men couldn't put Humpty Dumpty back together again."

A DIALECTICAL THEORY OF MIRRORING

As I (Seinfeld 1991b) discussed in a previous publication, Sartre focused on this negative side of mirroring. Although Winnicott described occasions of failure in mirroring, he emphasized its positive value in confirming the true self. Sartre saw mirroring as posing a dilemma. I must realize myself through the gaze of the other, but then my sense of self is defined by the other. I exist for myself in the mode of being for the other and discover myself as an object of the other. Sartre minimized the positive value of mirroring and instead underlined how mirroring objectifies the subject. It is from this comparison of Winnicott and Sartre and acceptance of their views that I propose the following dialectical theory of mirroring.

There is a need on the part of the infant to discover its sense of self through mirroring by the object. Mirroring initially confirms and reinforces an alive and vital sense of self, as described by Winnicott. The infant discovers itself in the mode of being for the other and experiences itself as captured in the reflection of the mirroring object (Seinfeld 1991b). It endeavors to escape from the object and recapture its sense of self. However, having lost the object, the infant experiences itself as alone, invisible, unseen, and unreal and is again in need of mirroring to confirm its being.

Although Winnicott conceived of mirroring in more positive terms than Sartre, there is nevertheless in his work an indication that he too recognized that the object poses intrinsic danger to the infant. Winnicott (1971b) spoke of the infant's need for contact and object relating but also an opposed need to remain incommunicado and inviolate. Here he refers to a secret self that needs to be protected from violation by the mother. It is necessary for the mother to be present to guard the child's potential space while he is alone, without intruding on him.

I think that the infant Winnicott speaks of as being object related is the self seeking mirroring, while the infant captured in the reflection of the mirror is the secret self demanding its autonomy. I am thereby conceiving of these selves not as static entities but as different opposing modes of functioning. Thus the infant's need for recognition followed by the effort to escape being captured in the reflection of the mirror is seen as a dialectical developmental process of alternating connection and separation. Jessica Benjamin (1988) has described development in terms of a dialectic tension between connection and separation. The child ideally experiences each cycle of recognition and separation on a higher level than the previous one as it becomes increasingly able to tolerate the anxieties associated with the need for recognition and the need to go unseen. The mother helps the child to negotiate the phases of recognition and escape. It is necessary to respond to the self needing recognition with excitement, interest, and awareness. It is necessary to respond to the secret self by remaining present but not intrusive, accepting rejection without retaliation, waiting patiently for the return of the child while guarding the potential space it plays in.

CLINICAL ASPECTS OF THERAPEUTIC REGRESSION

Winnicott described his views on therapeutic regression in the paper "Metapsychological and Clinical Aspects of Regression within the Psychoanalytic Set-Up" (1954). This study of regression was initiated by clinical work with patients who did not respond to the classical method. Analytic treatment is not merely a repertoire of techniques that the analyst administers to the patient. Winnicott emphasized that it requires a mastery of technique, which allows the analyst to be attuned to the process in which each patient follows his own particular pace. He divided patients into three categories. Those patients with intact personalities suffering from oedipal conflicts were treatable by classical analysis. The second group of patients, who have barely achieved wholeness of the personality and continue to be threatened by conflicts around love and hate, could be analyzed using the techniques of Melanie Klein. For such patients, Winnicott argued, interpretation is not the only curative factor. The patients' attacks on the analyst are often so intense that the outcome often rests on the analyst's capacity to survive these onslaughts. By this, Winnicott meant more than physical survival. He referred to the analyst's need to remain in empathic contact without retaliating or withdrawing. Therefore, with this second group of patients Winnicott introduces a holding function around management of negative countertransference in addition to the Kleinian method of interpretation.

The third group of patients, for whom personality structure is not securely formed, were open to treatment characterized as management. Here, the psychoanalyst must take up a holding function primarily because a patient has regressed to an early stage of development in which the mother's actual holding was necessary. The analysis must be focused on the most primitive stages of emotional development, before the attainment of personal unit status.

Along with Ferenczi and Balint, Winnicott found that some patients could undergo a classical analysis, intellectually understand in-depth interpretations, let go of symptoms, yet continue to feel that life was meaningless and futile. These patients had a tendency to regress to extreme levels of dependency. Winnicott described regression as the reverse of progress and the threat of chaos. He believed that it was normal for a person to defend the self against environmental failure by freezing the failure situation. Unconsciously, the patient assumed that there would be an opportunity at a later time for reliving the failure situation, which would then become unfrozen in an environment now making an adequate adaptive response. Winnicott believed that there was a biological drive toward progress that was set in motion by the unfreezing of the environmental failure situation. Regression was viewed as a healing process. Winnicott's view of regression as chaotic and the value of the therapist in tolerating it can be compared to the current scientific theory that says that chaotic phenomena have their own underlying order that strives toward higher levels of structure if left unhampered.

Winnicott believed that the third category of patients suffered very early trauma of the potential true self. A false-self organization took over and compliantly related to the maladaptive environment. A freezing of the failure situation is protected by the false self, but unfreezing can occur through regression. It is necessary in therapy to allow for primitive fusion states to let go of the false-self organization. The fusion or dependence is nearly absolute and is therefore primitive, disturbing, yet healing. The analytic session itself invites dependency by its reliability. Regression is a return to a need for early mothering in which the true self can meet environmental failures that are now limited in scope and therefore reliable.

HOLDING TECHNIQUES

Winnicott's holding efforts included extended sessions, telephone contacts, and sessions timed to accommodate a patient's needs. Margaret Little (1990) says that in wording interventions, Winnicott often spoke tentatively or speculatively. Interpretations were offerings that the patient was free to accept or reject. Winnicott would say, "I think perhaps . . ." or "I wonder if . . ." or "It seems to me as if . . ." rather than make an authoritative statement. He also practiced a technique described as revelation. Little, an analyst who had been analyzed by Winnicott, revealed that he helped her to become aware of the problems of her parents and her family life and their effect upon her. These interventions were more of a revelation than an interpretation because they helped her to face things she had always known but did not fully understand. Winnicott also utilized "explanation" to help the client understand how the horrific conditions the parent endured often accounted for the parent's maltreatment of the client. This explanation enabled the client to become less disposed to thinking that he was rejected because he was somehow intrinsically worthless.

Winnicott would express emotions that the patient had repressed or split off but were appropriate responses to environmental failure. In an analytic session, Winnicott asked Little why she always cried silently. She stated that once during her childhood she was crying from a toothache and was told to stop because she was making everyone unhappy. This made Winnicott very angry and he said that he hated her mother. On another occasion he expressed "shock" that the patient as a child had been forced to rest every afternoon in a darkened room with no toy or book.

Rayner (1991) reports that the technique used by both Winnicott and Balint that aroused the greatest indignation among classical analysts was an acceptance of the patient's need for physical contact, usually in the form of hand or head holding. There was never any concern about the ethical conduct of either analyst, but critics believed that actual holding must contain an element of eroticism. I would agree with the critics that, based on Fairbairn's view, libido is object seeking. As Rayner points out, the physical holding technique was a fashion of some forty years ago that did not stand the test of time.

Rayner (1991) states that Winnicott's technique of mirroring was quite similar to Carl Rogers's reflective techniques. Wright (1991b) says that language becomes purely symbol—an empty vehicle of meaning—only after the developmental process. The patient who remains at an early developmental level may use language more as a means of contacting a separate object than as a way to convey meaning. Words become something to throw back and forth, thereby making contact at a distance. Winnicott went beyond the model of therapy as work by describing therapy as play, even in the treatment of adults. In an earlier publication, I (Seinfeld 1991b) presented clinical vignettes illustrating the theme of schizoid patient captured in the reflection of mirroring. I will now provide examples of the holding function of mirroring.

FOUR CASE EXAMPLES

Example 1

A female patient had difficulty speaking but felt attacked or pressured if the therapist was active or engaging. She also became anxious if the therapist was silent. With time, she became better able to tolerate silence but more likely to feel attacked if the therapist spoke. She became silent for a good part of the session, and the therapist responded in kind. These near-silent sessions lasted for a few months. Winnicott has described how patients who were sensitive to intrusion needed to communicate that they wished to remain uncommunicative. The therapist in this case allowed the patient to use silence to express her desire not to communicate.

After this period, the patient expressed more of a readiness to speak, and the therapist became more active. The patient continued to be ambivalent about communicating, however, and ridiculed herself for not talking and for wasting her time and money. But if she spoke, she felt submissive. The therapist said, "You could make use of the session either by being silent or by speaking. Speaking is certainly an important part of therapy, but silence can also be of value. When you attack yourself for not communicating, does this facilitate communication?

> *Patient*: No. It only makes me feel badly about myself.
>
> *Therapist*: The purpose here is not to attack yourself but to understand what goes on when you speak or don't speak.
>
> *Patient*: That's different from how I ordinarily treat myself. I never try to understand, only to judge. Is it good or bad? More often than not it's bad and I attack. I don't know how to begin to understand.
>
> *Therapist*: If you speak only for the therapist, to be a good patient, this would not be authentic or good for you. If you were silent only to avoid difficulties—because you fear communication—silence will not help you to resolve the problem. If you are silent so that you can be with yourself—to be separate in my presence—this might be helpful. If you communicate as an authentic expression, this could be helpful.

In this session, the therapist endeavored to catalyze the patient to think by mirroring her dilemma while remaining neutral as to whether she should speak or remain silent. The therapist helped her play with possibilities to encourage autonomy.

The patient began to speak of dating. For months, when she was lonely and wishing for a man, no one took notice of her. Now, as she began to be independent and wished to be left alone, several men were interested in her.

It would be incorrect for the therapist to interpret that she feared intimacy would result in a loss of autonomy. Instead, the therapist might respond with exploration and mirroring. In this case, the therapist asked if she thought she had no wish to see men or if she felt some interest but was frightened. The patient replied that she thought she might enjoy being with the men but feared that her need for love would become intense and overwhelm her or that the men would make demands on her. The therapist then suggested that she perceived her own and/or the men's intense needs as a threat to her self-sufficiency. He asked if the men were, in fact, demanding. The patient thought about this for a moment but did not see any evidence of it. She suggested instead that because she was feeling very needy, she imagined that they were needy. She said that she wanted to be in a relationship but feared dependence. The therapist asked if she felt capable of managing both independence and a relationship. She replied that she was managing her own independence, so it was likely that she could manage a relationship as well. She could control the pace and level of involvement in a relationship.

The therapist stayed close to the patient's material, clarifying what she was saying or feeling and enabling her to arrive at her own interpretations. At some point, the therapist could interpret the totalization of conflict around intimacy and autonomy in the transference.

Example 2

A patient described the difficulty he was having completing a project. He reported that he was working on it every day and had achieved some progress, but had still not thrown himself into the work. However, he was trying to remain calm. The therapist replied that the patient's struggle to remain calm implied that he was trying to ward off a storm. This remark helped the patient to begin to explore the nature of his anxieties, whether the source was internal or external.

Shortly thereafter the patient described an admired friend who succeeded with a similar project. He described all of the unavoidable losses and tragedies that occurred throughout the friend's life. In describing how his friend now had a new position and was considerably better as a result of having completed the project, he said, "He suffered enough."

The therapist drew his attention to the curious phrase "suffered enough." The patient replied that it was just a figure of speech. The friend had suffered enough, so it was good that something positive had occurred. The therapist replied that the patient's wording could also suggest that the friend suffered enough so now something good could occur. The therapist did not insist on this meaning, only that the patient's words themselves suggested it. The patient then added, "Suffered enough so something good could occur, like in torment or guilt?" This led the patient to explore depressive position conflict, guilt, and its part in interfering with the completion of his own project.

The same patient described dating a woman who had kissed him goodnight on the corner where she lived instead of allowing him to walk her to her door. She had given some indication of liking him, but he felt rejected that she did not allow him to see her all the way home. He wanted to know what the therapist thought. The therapist responded by asking the patient what he thought. In the next session, the patient brought up the issue again, saying that he had felt rejected by the therapist for having turned the question back on him. The therapist now joined the patient more actively in looking at possible explanations as to why the woman did not want him to see her to the door. It was possible that she didn't like him, but there was concrete evidence to the contrary. It was possible that she thought he might ask and she didn't want to say no outright, fearing it would sour their developing relationship. It was also possible that she wanted him to come up to her apartment but feared he wouldn't ask. The patient then thought that his date had given some evidence of strongly valuing her independence and that she had wished to see herself to the door to stress her autonomy. It was also possible that her action didn't mean much at all.

Winnicott (1972) stressed that therapy could sometimes involve a "playing around" with ideas. As the patient played with these possibilities, he felt less rejected and more free to think. He began to wonder why he always jumped to the conclusion that he was being rejected. The holding technique therefore allowed the therapist to interpret the internal rejecting objects and conflicts around intimacy and sexuality.

Example 3

A severely disturbed patient said that she thought of moving out west and finding a job. She feared doing so because she might not find a job or a place to live, nor have any friends or money. The therapist replied that the patient thought of separating but feared that if she did so she would lose everything. This remark is an example of mirroring because the therapist here began to connect the patient's fear of separation with loss. It is not an interpretation because the therapist did not raise the issue of the patient's fear of being abandoned by an internal object if she separated.

The patient frequently described being stuck in situations that she disliked. She proved to be far from ready to make any changes in reality. The therapist's mirroring remarks can begin to help the patient see that being "stuck" is symptomatic of a fear of separation and loss.

Example 4

In his study of the mirror role, Winnicott (1971c) stated,

> When boys and girls in their secondary narcissism look in order to see beauty and to fall in love, there is always evidence that doubt has crept in about their mother's continued love and care. So the man who falls in love with beauty is quite different from the man who loves a [woman] and can see what is beautiful about her. [p. 113]

The patient described here in some ways fits Winnicott's description of the man who falls in love only with beauty.

The patient is a young adult working at a low-paying non-skilled job. However, he is beginning to improve by getting further job training and showing greater motivation. Familial stress and his own lack of self-assurance have delayed his development. He lives independently and is uncomfortable relating to women. Recently, he has made friends with several women but he feels unattractive and believes that the women will reject him.

He begins the session by remarking that he cannot establish a relationship.

Patient: It may be that when I meet a woman she's never good enough. I judge her by my friends' standards. I wonder if they would find her attractive. I think of them saying, "She's a real dog. What do you want with her?"

Therapist: So you see the woman through what you imagine to be your friends' eyes.

(The purpose here is not only to mirror the patient's remark but to illustrate that ultimately he is speaking of his own projection in describing his friends' standards.)

Patient: It's not really my friends but one friend, Ed.

Therapist: What about him—what is he about?

Patient: He's the one who has a different girl every night. And all of them are beautiful. It is his standard that I use.

Therapist: So you judge the women by what you think to be Ed's standard.

Patient: It's not really Ed's standard. He's a symbol. It's my standard.

Therapist: And what is that standard like and how does it work for you?

Patient: It annoys me. I wish it would leave me alone already. It puts me down. It says, "What is wrong with you? What do you want with her? Are you an idiot?" I can't stand it. After a while I say, "Stop it already."

Therapist: So you feel the standard to be oppressive, putting you down and restricting you. How does it work when you try to meet a woman? Does it help or hinder?

Patient: It never helps. If I meet a woman and I'm unsure if I'm interested, the standard disapproves. I never make any sexual innuendo because I don't want her to think I'm interested. It's as if my friend Ed is there warning me not to lead her on. She might take it the wrong way. I stop even being friendly. Sometimes women are responsive if I'm nice, and then this bell goes off.

Therapist: Let me just clarify. Is it that you have no interest in these women—or you're interested but the critical thoughts begin—or you're unsure.

Patient: At first, I feel an attraction. Then I'm unsure because of the standard. I think of two types of women. The women I've been discussing are ordinary. I mean regular women. The type I might meet at work, or in the neighborhood or at my new school. But then there's another type. I think of them as perfect and unattainable. I never made sexual allusions to them either. I imagined that because they were so perfect all men spoke to them of sex. I tried to be different, but they weren't interested. Then I changed my tactics and alluded to sexuality. That didn't work either. They were less interested. If I was simply friendly, they were more responsive.

Therapist: Could you say anything further about this second type?

Patient: They would be physically perfect. Women who could appear on the cover of *Vogue*. I believe it is women who select what type of woman appears on the cover because women read the magazine. Therefore, it is women who set the standard of beauty and men who take on that standard.

Therapist: So the standard that you said earlier was symbolized by your friend Ed is actually thought by you to be a woman's standard?

(The purpose here is to raise the possibility that the standard is actually from a woman in his history.)

Patient: Yes, I think it is a woman's standard.

Therapist: Then this standard doesn't help you with either type—the regular woman or the model.

Patient: I don't think I stand much of a chance with the *Vogue* type. I hardly earn a livable wage, and I'm only beginning to learn an employable skill. I can hardly take care of myself.

Therapist: The standard directs you toward a type you think you don't stand much of a chance with. It also discourages you from establishing a relationship with women you feel you might have a chance with.

Patient: I imagine it to be sitting on my shoulder and anytime I feel interested in someone, it whispers, "Not her—you can't." It reminds me of a television show. A man was surrounded by cockroaches in his home. They sang to him, "We love you, Joey, we always will. We'll be faithful, you know we will." That night, Joey was having a woman guest. He told the roaches to stay out of sight. They said they'd provide entertainment. He threw them a steak, begging them to disappear. He and the woman were having dinner and the roaches began to fall off the light fixture hung over their heads. The woman ran out. The roaches emerged singing, "We love you, Joey."

Therapist: (laughing) So the standard is a saboteur—it's like the cockroaches who love Joey and chase away the woman.

Patient: I'm recalling where the standard originated. I grew up with this very pretty girl, a friend of my family. I was attracted to her. It felt wrong—she was like a sister.

Therapist: So it felt incestuous?

Patient: Yes. The women who fit the perfect standard, the models—they're like her. I think they stand for her. She was not only beautiful but intelligent also. That's why my friend Ed's standard is only a symbol. His standard is quite low. Women only have to be good looking; he couldn't care less about their intelligence. Sometimes I'm like that. I don't care if they're nitwits. But I don't always feel that way.

The woman he imagines to set the standard for *Vogue* actually refers to the girl he grew up with. The perfect, unattainable image represents her. He has no sister, she is not his sister. Therefore, the incestuous feeling suggests she represents his mother, who is an incestuous object. He believes this type of woman finds him to be ugly. If this ideal female figure only looked upon him with acceptance, he imagines he would no longer feel ugly and worthless. The feeling of ugliness is likely to refer to an early failure of mirroring. There is also the incestuous taboo, but it is secondary to the theme of mirroring.

At first, this patient was not very communicative in treatment. He certainly did not free associate in the manner of a neurotic patient. The therapist's mirroring responses, however, elicited significant associations and memories. The therapist avoided interpretations and instead utilized reflection and clarification to facilitate communication. The patient drew closer to expressing interpretable material.

7

GUNTRIP, BION, STEWART, BOLLAS, JAMES, SAVEGE SCHARFF, WRIGHT, SEARLES, EIGEN, VOLKAN ON THE REGRESSED EGO

Harry Guntrip is largely responsible for popularizing Fairbairn's work in Great Britain and the United States. He provided a comprehensive and accessible presentation of Fairbairn's theories in his books *Personality Structure and Human Interaction* (1961) and *Schizoid Phenomena, Object Relations and the Self* (1969).

Guntrip was analyzed by both Fairbairn and Winnicott and integrated their work into what became known as the British middle school of object relations. He (1969) pointed out that Fairbairn's ego should more accurately be referred to as the self. Guntrip held that the self seeks cohesion and security through object relations. This is similar to Kohut's (1971) theory of the self object.

THE REGRESSED EGO

Guntrip extends Fairbairn's theory of endopsychic structure in a way that advanced the therapist's ability to provide a holding environment. He proposes a further splitting or subdivision of the already repressed libidinal ego into a withdrawn, regressed, and deadened self, where the ego is protected from the expected failures of external object relating. The libidinal ego is thus further divided into an orally active, sadomasochistic part, which continues to maintain internal bad object relations, and a passive regressed part, which seeks to return to the antenatal state of "absolute, passive, dependent security" (p. 74). I (Seinfeld 1990a) noted in an earlier publication that the regressed ego is a deficit state arising from failures in the infant caregiver relationship in which the infant did not feel loved as a person in its own right. Guntrip suggests that the tantalizing rejection of the exciting object probably results in the active sadomasochistic oral phenomenon, whereas impingement and deprivation give rise to the withdrawn, passive state. The regressed ego is described as a return to a symbolic womb. Guntrip says that security is established by phantasies of enclosure in a womblike state. Greenberg and Mitchell (1983) disagree with Guntrip's view, pointing out that even a symbolic womb implies a return to an object, possibly the phantasy of union with a perfect breast. However, Guntrip argues that there is a difference between womb, breast, and incest phantasies. He (1969) states,

> Womb fantasies cancel postnatal object relations; breast and incest fantasies do not. This fact makes an enormous difference to the ego, which is quite particularly dependent on object relationships for its strength and its sense of its own reality. Return to the womb is a flight from life and implies a giving up of breast and incest fantasies which involve a struggle to go on living. [p. 53]

I have found Guntrip's view of the regressed ego increasingly relevant in my work with the more advanced stages of transference and in regressions to the earliest stages of ego formation. I've noticed a general pattern in my work with several severe borderline patients. These patients would express overt rage when I went away for vacation during the first years of treatment. In this transference situation, the active sadomasochistic oral ego attacked the exciting but rejecting object, giving rise to depression and guilt. Throughout the middle phase of treatment, these patients were able to internalize enough of a positive image of the therapist to endure separation and to function more autonomously. Furthermore, the positive object relationship had grown strong enough to withstand a patient's rage. However, at a later phase of treatment, the patients

experienced a crisis state when they began struggling with becoming autonomous enough to separate from the objects who had
abandoned them throughout their lives. They suffered severe abandonment depression and terror, feeling that giving up bad objects
meant remaining isolated and never being able to establish good
object relationships.

A conflict arose over whether the regressed ego should be
allowed to emerge from withdrawal. The patients were in terror of
again experiencing the impingement, deprivation of object need,
and rejection that gave rise to the deepest and final split of the
libidinal ego. The relived the terror that originally led to the withdrawal of the regressed ego. At this point in the treatment, they
became exquisitely sensitive to any failure on the part of the therapist or other significant objects. Their situation represented a desperate vacillation between the regressed ego retreating from
disappointments that provoke the terror of reexperiencing early
object failure and the active oral sadomasochistic ego dreading
objectlessness and clinging to bad, persecutory objects.

Greenberg and Mitchell (1983) argue that Guntrip radically
departs from Fairbairn's basic theoretical premises. They read Guntrip as suggesting that the dread of objectlessness is the primary
motivating factor in seeking objects, whereas Fairbairn emphasized
the infant's object and reality relatedness from the beginning, before
there could be a dread of objectlessness. It is my sense that Greenberg and Mitchell overstate their case. Guntrip fully accepts Fairbairn's view that the infant is object related from the start. He
states, "In object-relational terms, the infant psyche is from the start
potentially an ego as yet undifferentiated as a structure, and it needs
a good enough human environment to make possible the actualiza-
tion of the ego through a developing process in object relations" (p.
386). The first anxiety is separation anxiety from the needed object.
For Fairbairn, there is a fear of objectlessness based on separations
or failures in relationship to the real external object. The infant at
the beginning is object seeking, but experiences of separation and
loss give rise to a fear of objectlessness, resulting in the internalization of the object. The tie to internal bad objects is based on the fear
of objectlessness; Fairbairn maintained that a bad object is better
than no object at all.

It is here that Guntrip's supplement to theory becomes relevant. The subject may be so persecuted by internal bad objects that there may be a further split, which gives rise to the regressed ego's retreat from internal persecutory objects. However, the subject has not entirely given up on object relations in that the active oral sadomasochistic libidinal self continues to struggle with the bad exciting and rejecting objects, allowing for the withdrawal of the regressed, passive self. Even the regressed, withdrawn self is not entirely removed from object relations in that it phantasizes a return to a symbolic womb. However, Guntrip insists on distinguishing between the quality of object relational phantasies with the breast and a return to the womb. The latter is technically still an object relationship. Thus Guntrip describes a simultaneous fight or flight reaction as the active sadomasochistic oral libidinal self struggles with internal objects and the regressed, passive self withdraws to phantasies of a return to the womb.

Mitchell and Greenberg argue that Guntrip bases the need for objects on the dread of objectlessness. Guntrip says that the withdrawn, regressed self exerts an attraction of the remaining personality. There is a regressive pull away from unsatisfactory and undermining object relations toward a protective, withdrawn regressed state. However, the regressive pull results in a fear of objectlessness, which in turn gives rise to a clinging to internal and external objects. Guntrip never claims that this dread of objectlessness gives rise to the original need for objects. Rather, he describes a secondary defensive need for objects on the part of schizoid personalities after a prolonged development of splitting and regressions.

REACHING THE REGRESSED, WITHDRAWN EGO

Guntrip's theoretical views led him to believe that the analyst must provide a holding function to reach the regressed ego. The therapist must be a good enough object in reality so that the withdrawn ego can emerge from the symbolic womb. In effect, it is necessary for the therapist to breach the closed system of internal bad objects in order to reach the lost, withdrawn, and lonely self of the patient. Guntrip believes that the patient who phantasizes about a return to a symbolic womb may also experience a psychic rebirth. He emphasizes the importance of the therapist's reaching out to the patient. Guntrip (1969) describes a patient dreaming that she is lost on one side of a river. In the dream she is watching a man on the other bank who can only reach her by crossing over. Guntrip interprets that he is the man in the dream who must somehow find a way to reach the patient's regressed ego because she cannot reach out to him.

In my own clinical experience, I have encountered schizoid patients who are likely to avoid sessions and not call for help, no matter how distressed. Such patients are unable to ask for help, and it may be necessary for the therapist in such situations to initiate action.

Another technique I utilize with such patients is tracking their awareness of the therapeutic relationship between sessions. Patients may have no sense of an inner relationship to sustain them when faced with the absence of an actual object. George Frank (personal communication 1980) originated the technique of helping a patient become aware of deficits, such as an inability to evoke a remembrance of a positive object relationship with which to comfort himself. The patient cannot try to correct such a deficit until he becomes aware of it. I (Seinfeld 1990a) described this technique in an earlier publication.

Efforts to reach out to the patient must be done with caution, appropriate timing, and respect for the patient's autonomy. Winnicott (1962) cautioned that the schizoid patient is vulnerable to impingement and needs the analyst to be present but not imposing. Only after the therapist has convincingly demonstrated that he supports the patient's autonomy can he usefully reach out, even then only sparingly and when fully warranted.

Wilfred Bion

In Chapter 3, I described Kleinian technique in terms of the paternal function of interpretation. Actually, there is a maternal function in Kleinian technique that was introduced by Wilfred Bion.

Bion (1962) viewed the infant–mother relationship as the prototype of the analyst's containing function. The infant projects unwanted parts of its psyche into the mother. The mother (or good breast) contains the infant's projected bad feelings by engaging in a state of reverie. She metabolizes the infant's disowned self-states, and the infant reintrojects the bad but now manageable feelings. The mother's maternal function enables the negative feelings to become manageable for the infant. If the caregiver is overwhelmed by the infant's anxiety, she may distance herself. She deprives the infant of the containing function in which she tolerates her own signal anxiety and returns to a calm state, thereby quieting the infant.

Bion maintained that the analyst performs a similar containing function for the patient. The analyst is receptive to the patient's projections by freeing himself, before each session, of memory, understanding, and desire.

A patient I treated described how she had seen a previous therapist when she was at great risk of abusing her child. He required her to put her murderous feelings into words but not act on them. She did so and credited his efforts with saving both herself and her child. Not only did the therapist allow her to ventilate her feelings but he tolerated feelings she could barely manage, remaining calm and concerned but not overwhelmed. The patient thought of him as being dependable and identified with his strength. His recommendation that she put her feelings into words but not act on them is an example of the paternal function, while his receptivity to her projections and management of his own feelings are examples of the maternal containing function.

There are schizoid and schizophrenic patients who evidence an incapacity to utilize projection and projective identification. I think that Bion's views can be extended to explain this phenomenon. For the patient to employ projection, there must be the idea of an object to receive and contain the projections. Therefore, it is likely that schizoid patients suffer from a deficit or lack of an internal containing object. The holding function of the therapist would therefore be the establishment of an internal containing object. Chapters 12, 13, and 14 will describe through clinical vignettes how the therapist fulfills this function.

RECENT CONTRIBUTIONS ON
THERAPEUTIC REGRESSION

The theme of benign regression occurs throughout the writings of many recent authors of the British and American object relations traditions. Rayner (1991) defines benign regression as characterized by a state of undifferentiation between self and object. Little (1986) describes therapeutic regression in her work on basic unity. She emphasizes that certain schizoid patients may only focus on reality to defend against a delusional transference of merger with the analyst.

Both Balint and Winnicott described patients with very severe pathology. The emphasis today, however, is on patients who only partially operate on a false-self basis. In fact, everyone may experience certain aspects of functioning that can be described as "basically faulted." This attitude accords well with Fairbairn's view of the schizoid position as universal. This implies that regression is an aspect in every therapeutic experience. Winnicott believed that there would be moments of regression to earliest dependency in all analysis. Rayner (1991) maintains that not every patient needs the extensive regressions described by Balint and Winnicott. A patient may experience regression within the boundary of the session to move out of it, understanding and leaving it. Kris's (1952) regression in the service of the ego may be the ideal.

Harold Stewart

Stewart (1986) provides a contemporary reconsideration of Balint's work addressing the level of the basic fault. He recommends that the therapist avoid directing all interpretations to the transference early in treatment, a trend associated with the Kleinian view. According to Stewart, the analyst's assuming an omnipotent position enhances the danger of malignant regression. Stewart also cautions that interpretations of sexual fantasies or conflicts when the patient is regressed to the level of the basic fault can evoke states of overexcitement or overstimulation, which can result in malignant regression.

Christopher Bollas

Bollas (1987) aptly describes benign regression. The patient, un-aware of the analyst's presence, falls into a twilight state and attends to lying on the couch, listening to the passing cars or the ticking of the clock. There is a subtle redirection of attention from the outside world to the inside. This is viewed as an intermediate area of experience: the patient is between reception and evocation. The patient then recalls a dream or a memory, something he never thought but always knew, that he now wishes to tell the analyst. Thus, for Bollas, benign regression results in a loosening of attention and thought to the intermediate space that evokes meaningful associations.

Martin James

James (1985) describes the infant's lacking of a good enough holding environment. He emphasizes that the aspect of the holding environment he considers is that of the caregiver's continual presence and empathy through which she can anticipate and avert overstimulation that could overwhelm the baby. On the basis of his studies, James finds that the infant lacking in a good enough holding environment may give the impression of a much older baby, as it had to develop prematurely the capacity to screen out noxious stimulus, to anticipate environmental reactions, and to tolerate delays of gratification. The infant experienced premature ego development during the first months of life by taking over functions the caregiver failed to perform. Thus, as I described in the discussion of Guntrip's work, the infant develops a barrier to protect itself from impingement. In warding off impingement from the object world, the child also deprives itself of the opportunity to internalize an ideal object. Patients who suffered this early failure by the holding environment are likely to develop the regressed ego described by Guntrip.

Jill Savege Scharff

Scharff (1992) points to "the forgotten concept of introjective identification" (p. 67). As she notes, analytic literature has focused

significantly more attention on projective than on introjective identification. Scharff differentiates between introjection and incorporation. In describing the transposition of the external object into the
subject, she states, "To my mind, however, a distinction between
introjection and incorporation could be made: In introjection the
transposition is achieved by receptiveness without the accompa-
nying fantasy of the object's penetration that is characteristic [of]
the process of incorporation" (p. 82). Also, introjection refers to the
transposition of objects into the psychic apparatus—the ego or the
ego ideal. Introjection does not have the same lateral correlation
with the actual body as does incorporation. Thus Scharff's use of
the term *introjection* strongly resembles the American ego psychological notion of object constancy, which emphasizes the internalization of a positive or libidinal object representation within the
ego. In introjective identification the subject's ego then becomes
similar to that of the object. This is different from projective identification, in which the object's ego becomes similar to that of the
subject.

This emphasis on introjective identification advances the
holding function of the psychotherapist. Scharff describes the therapeutic value in the patient's introjection of the therapist as an ideal
object. She describes a patient called Mrs. Findley who had under-
gone years of therapy for suicidal ideation, poor self-esteem, depression, and rages at her children. The patient had been sexually
and violently abused by her alcoholic, suicidal mother. She had
seemingly adored her father but then became aware of her rage at
him for not protecting her from the abuse. In fact, the only person
she received loving mothering from was her maternal grandmother. Scharff describes how the patient first transferred onto her
the idealizing transference toward the maternal grandmother, also
creating her in the form of the ideal mother she lacked. Scharff says,

> Mrs. Findley's capacity for introjective identification with the
> ideal object promoted a degree of ego strength that militated
> against the inevitability of a borderline personality structure. Her
> introjective identification with me as such an ideal object as her
> grandmother functioned as an effective and necessary defense
> against the reentry of the projective identification of me as a

harmful mother object that had been split-off in analysis as it had
been in childhood. [p. 61]

Scharff accepted the patient's idealization without prematurely interpreting splitting, allowing for the internalization of the
ideal object. Only after the defense and resistance were sufficiently
strengthened did she interpret how the ideal grandmother transference defended against the abandoning and abusive mother transference. I would add to Scharff's analysis that by accepting the
idealizing transference, she not only strengthened a defense but
catalyzed the growth of a psychic structure—that of the ideal object.

As Scharff points out, Fairbairn believes that introjection underlies all psychic structure. The inevitable failures of even good
mothering give rise to the need to take in and control the object.
Scharff notes how Fairbairn is less vivid in his description of good
aspects of internal object relationship as he focused on how the
good object was split off to protect it from its bad counterparts.
Scharff adds that she revised her view as she later read Fairbairn as
saying that good object experience is secondarily introjected to fill
the psychic void. As can be seen in Chapter 4 in this volume, I read
Fairbairn in much the same way. However, as I remarked earlier, he
still does not sufficiently attend to the development of the internal
good object through introjective identification. His technique involves interpreting the split-off bad objects so that they can be
integrated with the ideal object. At the same time, he acknowledges
that interpretation is secondary to the quality of the therapeutic
object relationship.

I believe that now the full implications of Fairbairn's views can
be explicated. Interpretations that attempt to integrate the ideal and
bad internal objects will result in the ideal object being overwhelmed and subsumed by the bad objects if it is insufficiently
developed. For this reason, it was essential for Scharff to shore up
the introjective identification of the ideal object of her patient Mrs.
Findley before proceeding to interpret the splitting that protected
the ideal object and idealized transference from the bad objects.
Mrs. Findley had begun to develop an ideal object on the basis of a
grandmother who provided her with loving mothering. Therefore,
the ideal object could be strengthened by the analyst accepting and

empathizing with the transference. However, if the patient did not experience good mothering from anyone in reality, it might be necessary for the therapist to take a more active stance in the form of reaching out as described by Guntrip (1969).

Kenneth Wright

For Wright (1991b), the unconscious is the place where the mother is not; it is outside both her vision and her love. It is the mother's vision that brings structure to the infant's world. All that she rejects or that the child does not let her see becomes the unconscious.

Wright (1991b) presents an important theory of symbol formation that tracks symbol development from things to meaning. The first symbol is the transitional object. Since the baby cannot yet separate meaning from its representation, the transitional object serves as an embodiment or incarnation. There is a transference of the softness or sensory pattern of the mother to a blanket or some other object. The infant becomes capable of matching the sensory pattern of the mother with a similar sensory pattern in the world surrounding it. Meaning cannot yet be held in the infant's consciousness in a detached or abstracted form or representation. There must be at first a fleeting sense of separateness that leads to tolerance of separateness, which in turn results in a holding off from the object supported by vision.

Wright describes how a symbol (unconscious) in dreams or in symptoms still exists as an exclusively carnal mode embodying an undiscovered meaning. At this point, the child is in the mode of acting and doing and is not yet able to be separate. Holding off is only experienced in the physical mode. The unconscious symbol is imaginary, not imagined. In my earlier discussions of Abraham and Fairbairn, I illustrated how the individual might live and suffer a psychological situation so that he remains unaware of feelings expressed through a symbolic displacement but felt in a real way. For instance, the breast, feces, urine, phallus, and internal part-objects are such unconscious symbols. The patient is used by the symbol instead of using the symbol. The dream or symptom—unconscious symbols—are enactments, not communications.

Wright separates such unconscious symbols from fully developed symbols that become hollow metaphors, transparencies, and
space for meaning. A fully developed symbol implies accepting its
nonreal status, separating representation from the thing itself represented, substituting looking for doing, and viewing the self from
the outside, the position of the third in the oedipal dyad. Arriving at
the fully developed symbol means living within the symbolic order
where the world is structured through language and ideologies,
religions, self-images, and worldviews.

Wright draws on Winnicott's idea of transitional phenomena
to distinguish the transitional object from play. In the transitional
object the pattern of the mother is found in the single object and no
other. In play, however, the pattern is recognized in itself and can be
transferred from object to object. Wright (1991b) describes how the
freeing of the pattern from the object is a momentous discovery for
the child. When the child wanted the pattern earlier, he was at the
mercy of the object that contained it: "The freeing of the pattern
frees the child from this bondage. He possesses the pattern, and can
now use it for his own purposes" (p. 249).

With this possession of the pattern, the child can now perpet-
uate on its own the original maternal function of providing presence
and comfort. Through play and merger experiences, the comforting
feel of the mother and the pattern of interaction between infant and
mother are carried over into the world-other-than-mother, thereby
supporting separation. Drawing on the views of Suzanne Langer,
Wright distinguishes presentational symbolism, which deals with
play, music, and art, from discursive symbolism, which involves
language, logic, and pure abstract representation.

It may now be seen that the presentational symbol is the
expression of the maternal function, whereas the discursive symbol
is related to the paternal function. The presentational symbol is
usually nonverbal and presents directly, whereas the discursive
symbol is verbal and refers to the thing represented.

An examination of Martin Buber's I-you and I-it relations
may help to further clarify the maternal and paternal functions. (See
also Chapter 10.) For Buber (1958), the I-you relation is direct,
immediate, and supports and encounters being. It refers to the
intersubjective being of two entities. The I-it relation is analytic,

objectifies, and attempts to talk about and to take apart the it into its constituent parts: "It has created the crucial barrier between subject and object; the basic word I-it, the word of separation, has spoken" (p. 75).

Buber (1958) emphasizes that both the I-you and the I-it are essential ways of relating to the world. The I-you provides a foundation of being and can be referred to as the maternal function. The I-it provides a sense of doing and separateness and can be referred to as the paternal function. For doing and separation to be authentic, they must rest on a solid foundation of being.

Harold Searles

Harold Searles is one of the most influential and creative analysts in advancing the importance of the holding relationship. He (1965) described four phases of patient–therapist interaction in the treatment of severely disturbed patients. In the initial out-of-contact phase, the patient and therapist are isolated in their own psychic territories and the therapist must find a nonintrusive way to enter the patient's world. In the ambivalent symbiotic phase, the patient and therapist recapitulate the modes in which the patient and his parents drove one another crazy through projective and introjective identification. It is the third phase—therapeutic symbiosis—that is the clearest expression of the maternal function. Searles emphasized that during this crucial period the therapist and patient are just being together and not doing to one another, thereby allowing the patient the opportunity to be without impingement. In the fourth and final phase, resolution of symbiosis, Searles refined some of Ferenczi's most important ideas. It will be recalled that Ferenczi experimented with mutual analysis between patient and analyst and described how the patient remained loyal and altruistic toward the abusive parent. Searles described how the patient projects the pathogenic parental object onto the therapist, inducing the therapist to experience the conflicts, feelings, and behavior of the original parent. The patient often finds something in the actuality of the therapist's personality to serve as a fitting container for the internal object. Like Ferenczi, Searles noted how the parent of the patient somehow communicated to the child a need for help. The child endeavored to help the parent not only out of altruism but also out of a desire to make the parent into a better parent to meet the child's innate need for ego care. However, although the parent sought the child's help, the parent had an equally strong need to defeat the child's effort. This caused the child to experience himself as a failed therapist. Searles's (1975) most important innovation involves suggesting that the patient continues to act out the need to both re-create and cure the crazy parent. The patient will either induce the therapist to fail him or be astute to failings on the part of the therapist. The patient will then endeavor to help the therapist overcome his failings and cure the crazy parent in the transference. The difference between the original object and the therapist is that the latter may be more successful then the original parent in making use of the patient's efforts.

Harold Searles was among the first American analysts to describe projective and introjective identifications in the transference–countertransference situations. His papers on schizophrenia in the 1960s discussed British object relations theorists, who were in turn influenced by his pioneering work.

Michael Eigen

Michael Eigen is another pioneering analyst who has made important contributions to the holding relationship theory. He (1980) described the significance of the human face in healthy infant development in terms similar to Kenneth Wright's work. Eigen also discussed the theories of Winnicott, Lacan, and Sartre concerning this issue. He agreed with Spitz that the infant stared at the mother's face, not her breast, and that it was visual stimulation and not oral tactile sensation that triggered the smiling response in the infant. However, Eigen took issue with Spitz that the smiling response could be accounted for wholly in terms of its functional value of eliciting empathic maternal responses in the mother to ensure the infant's survival. He emphasized instead that the smiling response always took place at a certain distance, did not arise by touch alone, was visual, and was an important part of the interplay between closeness and distance that defined self- and other awareness. Eigen stated that he understood the smiling response not primarily in terms of a nonintentional but manipulative biological signal but rather in terms of "an expression of alive and vibrant delight" (p. 56). Here Eigen also distinguishes the difference between Winnicott and Spitz's views of the infant's relation to the mother's face. Although both recognize its importance, Winnicott's emphasis is on the mirroring and actualizing of existence, whereas Spitz's focus remains biological and ultimately refers to the gratification of instinctual drives and a signal support to aid survival. Eigen suggested that his clinical experience led him to believe that the human face is experienced as self yet other. There is a subject-to-subject reality in which the human face is experienced in its aliveness. I consider the subject-to-subject original relationship as synonymous with Martin Buber's I-you relation. It is the failures in the subjectivity-subjectivity relation that give rise to the need to possess, devour, or know the other as an it or an object.

Eigen found that the recognition of the mother's face indicates that another personality is present. It is in the presence of the mother that the infant's being is affirmed. Eigen made the important suggestion that in the face of panic over the absence of the mother, it is likely that the mother's face and not her breast is remembered for comfort. In my view, an important implication of this idea is that the severely disturbed patient lacking in object constancy may sometimes need face-to-face sessions to facilitate the internalization of the analyst's face.

Referring to Guntrip's (1969) concept of the passive, regressed ego, Eigen (1973) pointed out that this ego structure is active and alive in its passivity and density. Drawing on the views of Elkin, Eigen referred to the regressed ego as the *schizoid ego*, an aspect of self that retreats to a detached, hidden existence. It seems to me that it is the internalization of what Eigen referred to as the "glowing face" of the maternal object that can warm and enliven the withdrawn or schizoid ego.

Vamık Volkan

Volkan (1987) says that in America there tend to be two styles of treatment with preoedipal patients. The first view discourages regression and attempts to support the patient at the level at which he can function while providing new ego experiences to enable him to integrate opposing self- and object images. Therapists oriented to this style believe that the already severely disturbed patient will become psychotic or act out. Volkan includes Knight, Zetzel, Wallerstein, and Kernberg among these therapists. For them there is considerable concern about the role of innate pregenital aggression and the possibility of its reaching unmanageable proportions.

The proponents of the second style believe that patients need to regress to a lower level than the current chaotic one. Regression allows patients to progress through healthier developmental levels, as children do in a good enough holding environment. Advocates of this second approach emphasize that a patient may need to relive early experiences of deprivation and environmental failure in an intense transference situation. In fact, the patient may relive a full symbiotic relatedness that allows for a new separation-individuation experience in relation to the therapist. The British view of the holding relationship and therapeutic regression is synonymous with the American idea of therapeutic symbiosis. Among American analysts who advocate therapeutic regression are Bryce Boyer, Harold Searles, Peter Giovacchini, Michael Eigen, and Vamık Volkan. All of them have had considerable long-term intensive analytic experience with psychotic patients and favor allowing the patient to undergo regression to a psychotic transference to effect structural change. I am in agreement with this group. The idea of psychotic transference is synonymous with the British view of the patient experiencing a harmonious mix-up or undifferentiated state between self and object in the transference situation.

Loewald (1960) stated that the analyst validates the patient's regressive experience as genuine by having a corresponding therapeutic regression of his own so as not to leave the patient all alone with his. He likened the therapeutic regression to the involvement of the parent in the parent-child relationship. The therapist's emotional involvement in the care of the patient creates a dyad similar in intensity to that of the early infant-mother unit. The therapist's regression should remain controlled and in the service of the ego and the other. It should involve experiencing primary therapeutic preoccupation during crucial points in the treatment, being receptive to trying on the patient's projections, and remaining emotionally available to the patient in accord with his developmental needs.

8

THE IDEAL OBJECT AND THE REGRESSED SELF

THE DEFICIT IN AN INNER IDEAL OBJECT AND BAD OBJECTS

In an earlier publication I (Seinfeld 1991a) described how the lack of love is experienced as a psychic hunger based on physiological emptiness. The inevitable failures of loving on the part of the caregiver give rise to an empty core in the infant, or a hunger to incorporate part-objects. For Fairbairn, good objects were internalized only as a defense against bad objects. This view neglects the importance of the internal good object in assisting the infant in separating from external objects and in contributing to psychic structure. Fairbairn does not provide sufficient discrimination between internal good objects that serve purely defensive purposes and those that serve adaptation. Furthermore, he described the ideal good internal object as being projected onto external objects, a view that did not allow for a full elaboration of the ideal object as experienced on the inside and in relationship to bad objects. The projection of the ideal object onto the external object world leaves the patient's inner world void of the experience of a good object. I propose that the already repressed libidinal ego splits off into the withdrawn, regressed ego (Guntrip 1969) because of the lack of a good internal object.

The good or ideal internal object is based on actual loving and caring experiences in the infant–mother relationship. If this relationship is unsatisfactory, there will be a deficiency of an internal good object. In a previous publication I (Seinfeld 1990a) discussed how the regressed ego is a deficit state. The regressed ego remains in a deficit state because the internal good object, to which it is attached libidinally, is also in a deficit state. Furthermore, the regressed ego is divided from the internal good object because the latter is either attacked and expelled by bad internal objects or projected onto external objects to protect it from bad objects.

Scharff and Scharff (1992) feel that Fairbairn implies that the normal or mature ideal object is identical with the ideal object of the schizoid or hysteric patient devoid of libidinal excitement or aggression. On other occasions, Fairbairn suggests that the central self strives for the integration of split-off self and object components, implying that a split-off ideal object completely void of exciting or aggressive qualities would not be the norm. In my view, the radical splitting off of the ideal object from any exciting or aggressive qualities is the result of the deficiency of the ideal object, which is weakened and therefore in danger of being overwhelmed if integrated with exciting or rejecting bad objects. The splitting and projection of the ideal object of the schizoid or hysteric patient is therefore a desperate effort to protect the weak, deficit ideal object from being overwhelmed or expelled by the split-off bad objects. Premature interpretation of splitting would be counterproductive because the ideal object could not withstand the bad objects. However, the protective projection and splitting off of the ideal object leave the libidinal ego without the support of an inner good object and cause the further splitting of the already repressed libidinal ego into the withdrawn ego described by Guntrip (1969). If the good inner object is overwhelmed or anally expelled by the antilibidinal self or rejecting object, the patient is left with a further sense of emptiness.

Fairbairn (1958) said that the essential therapeutic task was to cause a breach in the patient's closed system of inner reality. I would add that the therapist must help the patient establish a good internal object in the transference to reach the regressed ego to allow it to emerge in attachment to an internal good object. Kleinians such as Herbert Rosenfeld (1987) described the persecution of the ideal object by persecutory bad objects. Rosenfeld refers to this phenomenon in terms of destructive narcissism that attacks the dependent self or positive libidinal object relationships. The destructive and omnipotent aspects of the psyche are often disguised, split off, or silent and play a powerful role in preventing or devaluing good object relationships. Patients may appear to be indifferent to the external object world. They may feel that they have given life to themselves and are able to meet all of their own needs. They may prefer to die, deny the fact of their birth, and destroy any potential for help rather than depend on the analyst. Self-destructive acting out may be idealized as an answer to their problems. Rosenfeld distinguishes between narcissism that is healthy and provides libidinal enhancement of the self and narcissism that causes an idealization of destructive aspects of the self. He believes that destructive narcissism is a manifestation of the death instinct, which finds expression in a chronic paralysis that keeps the patient from living, prompts intense anxiety about dying, and opposes the patient's will to live. Rosenfeld finds that the death force becomes more deadly and threatening when the patient turns more toward life and good sustaining objects.

Fairbairn recognized the clinical phenomena attributed to the death instinct; however, he rejected this explanation and instead asserted that the patient was trapped within a closed psychic system of bad objects based on early unsatisfactory relationships with significant external objects. He emphasized an obstinate tendency on the patient's part to keep both aggression and libido localized within the confines of the inner world as a closed system because of a sense of hopelessness about obtaining satisfaction in relationships with significant external objects.

What I am suggesting is that the patient's antilibidinal ego may identify with the rejecting object and attack the internal good object. This is an idea that I (Seinfeld 1990a) put forth elsewhere in describing the negative therapeutic reaction, which I now see as significant for most cases of failed object constancy. The potential good object is quick to become an overly exciting object because the libidinal self's dependency needs have remained primitive and have grown even more intense. Frustration or the original external object at first provided comfort and ego care but then became overly stimulating and engulfing. There may be cases in which the exciting object is so radically divorced from the good object that it works in the service of the rejecting object by luring the libidinal self into destructive addictions as opposed to good human object relationships.

The most crucial consideration is that the regressed, withdrawn, deadened self is split off from its potential attachment to the deficient internal good object. An ideal object that is utterly devoid of exciting and aggressive aspects will not be vital or real enough to enliven and reach the regressed self. The therapist must provide a real holding environment so as to be internalized not as a schizoid ideal object but as an alive and caring object. It is to be expected that the patient will resort to a degree of idealization to protect the good internal object from the antilibidinal self. The therapist interprets the attacks of the antilibidinal self and the rejecting object on the internalization of the good object. If the therapist prematurely interprets the defensive idealization and splitting of the good object, integration could result in the deficient and weakened good object being overwhelmed by the stronger bad objects. Only after the good object is strengthened by the holding environment should the therapist provide interpretations to effect integration. The patient may need a prolonged period of introjecting and identifying with the analyst as an ideal object before he can tolerate integrating the ideal object with the split-off exciting and rejecting transferential objects.

The following clinical vignettes will illustrate how the internal persecutory objects attack the vulnerable libidinal self's need for the ideal object.

CASE EXAMPLES

Example 1

Isaac, a bright, articulate, religious Jewish man in his early forties, was referred to me through a Jewish mental health clinic. He described himself as feeling schizophrenic. When I explored this, he revealed suffering from clinical depression throughout his life. He was on antidepressant medication but thought that it was no longer effective. He felt confused, indecisive, saying he did not know if he was "coming or going."

Isaac grew up in an intact family with three siblings. His parents were Holocaust survivors, and most of his extended family had died in the war. His father was a complex, histrionic man. Isaac felt that he took after his father. He described his mother as a highly critical but simple, down-to-earth woman. In fact, both parents were domineering, guilt inducing, and threatened by their children's attempts to lead their own lives. He felt that their fears were partially the result of the losses suffered from the Holocaust.

Isaac was married with one child. A businessman, he could not concentrate on his work and rarely went to the office. His only enjoyment consisted of studying the Talmud with an older man. His partner in talmudic studies believed that Isaac demonstrated an unusually good understanding of the texts. However, Isaac was typically too depressed to pursue his studies with regularity.

Isaac presented contemporary family problems. His latency-aged son Reuben was depressed and hyperactive, and functioned poorly in school. Isaac overidentified with Reuben and sometimes overprotected him. He sometimes permitted Reuben to sleep with his wife and him, to miss school, and to buy whatever he wanted. Isaac described his wife as intelligent but emotionally aloof. She had suffered emotional deprivation throughout childhood and therefore had difficulty giving of herself. She was sometimes overwhelmed in caring for Reuben, who was a difficult child. Despite their emotional problems, they were both committed to providing Reuben with the help and care he needed.

Throughout our sessions, Isaac repeatedly complained of how tortured he felt. He said that his heart pounded, he was exhausted, he could not think straight, and he might collapse at any moment. He rarely discussed what was going on emotionally or in his personal life that contributed to his feeling so distraught.

It was necessary for me to balance holding and interpretation. If I focused only on Isaac's symptoms, he avoided the underlying issues. However, if I immediately tried to explore underlying issues, he felt that I was unwilling to contain his troubled feelings. Therefore, for a number of sessions I just sat and listened. Finally, I said, "You describe how badly you feel. This is very important. However, your distressing emotional and physical states are the end result of emotional and personal problems. The focus on the pain of your symptoms sometimes allows you to ignore the personal dimension."

Isaac expressed curiosity about what I had in mind and I said, "Personal problems often reflect problems with significant people or your feelings about those people or yourself. The pain is important in its own right, and you will often need to discuss it, but when you focus exclusively on it, you may be diverting yourself from looking at the underlying personal and emotional issues."

Isaac sometimes said the pain was too severe to cope with. He could not believe he would ever get better. I emphasized that therapy takes time and patience, that when he was trapped with his distressing feelings he could not picture himself ever feeling differently. He had had these problems his entire life, so they would not be alleviated quickly.

During one session he said, "It was very strange when I woke up the other day."

> *Therapist*: How so?
> *Isaac*: I felt good. For the first time I could remember. Not schizophrenic, not depressed.
> *Therapist*: Yes?
> *Isaac*: I had this thought. I feel good. I'm not tormented. I was aware of this. Then I wondered for how long I would feel good. When would it end? Then the next thing I knew, it was back—misery again.
> *Therapist*: So you were feeling good and wondering how long it would last and that was the end of it. Almost as if you were warning yourself. Time to stop feeling good—it's been going on for too long. You are not allowed.
> *Isaac*: It's crazy. It felt like that. Not only did I get depressed, I was more depressed than usual. It was as if something inside said, "So you want to feel good. You think you can feel good. You want trouble. I'll give you trouble."

Over the next several weeks, Isaac became aware of a force that threatened to beat him down whenever there was the possibility of feeling better. Feeling paralyzed, suffering, behaving self-destructively were now understood as expressions of this negative force. He realized that his negative thoughts about areas in his life that were realistically problematic—his marital problems, his son's problems, the lack of direction in his life—were utilized to depress and defeat him. I helped him to become aware of this by first asking, "Where do these self-criticisms go? What do they lead to? Do they bring about any change?"

Isaac replied, "No, it's the opposite. They paralyze me. I feel overwhelmed. Everything seems hopeless."

> *Therapist*: Therefore these thoughts seem to be expressions of this destructive force that exploits realistic problems in an effort to paralyze or depress you. It sounds like an internal parent relentlessly telling you all that is wrong.
> *Isaac*: When this occurs I feel like a slave being beaten. I want to liberate myself from this cruel taskmaster. How do I do it?

Shortly thereafter, Isaac likened the therapy to the tale of Moses. He said that the therapist is like God telling him, Moses, to go before Pharaoh, his internal tyrant, and say, "Let my people go."

Pharaoh laughs and says, "You think you can tell me what to do. You think you can go free. I'm the only one who gives orders. I'll show you."

The inner Pharaoh tortures him with plagues, torments. Isaac as Moses runs to the therapist as God and asks what to do. God says, "Go back; tell him, let my people go." So he does, but the internal tyrant says, "You're back. So you want trouble. This time I'll show you. Now you're going to get it."

After recounting this story, Isaac laughed, saying, "This is what it's like. I'm between you and this inner tyrant. But I guess the idea is to stick with it. The story concludes with Moses and the Israelites being freed from Egypt. They cross the Red Sea and Pharaoh's troops drown in pursuit. Are you going to deliver me to the Promise Land? I guess you do in the end."

Therapist: If I recall the story, it doesn't go so smoothly. After fleeing from Egypt, Moses and the Israelites struggle on in the desert for what seems like forever. They struggle with themselves and with God. In fact, I think Moses never reaches the Promised Land, although he gets close.

Isaac: Yes. So maybe that means there's a long, arduous road ahead—I might not even achieve all that I wish for—but what I achieve will help my people, that is, my family. Maybe it's my child who will reach the Promised Land.

Reuben, Isaac's son, suffered from depression and severe anxiety, and had been in special class placement and therapy throughout the year. Over the last few months, Isaac had forced Reuben to attend school each day despite the child's anxiety and wish to stay at home. Now Isaac decided to send the boy away to summer camp for the first time. At first, Reuben was ambivalent about going to camp, but then, to Isaac's surprise, he agreed to it. Isaac now experienced much trepidation about whether his son would manage away from home for a month. He felt that it would be a miracle if Reuben stayed for the entire term.

Reuben went and enjoyed camp. Isaac then wondered if Reuben might remain for the entire summer instead of only the month of July. Reuben showed signs of being stressed by the new experience, and the camp officials felt it was better for him to return home as originally planned and thereby have a successful experience. Isaac was disappointed that Reuben did not remain for the entire summer.

In August, the family stayed at a house in the country. In the past, Reuben had slept late in the morning but had gone in the afternoon to a local day camp. By sleeping late, he missed the morning session at camp.

Isaac came into a therapy session angry. He was going to lay down the law with Reuben. Now that Reuben had proved himself by attending sleep-away camp, Isaac expected him to leave for day camp early in the morning. He was no longer going to be indulgent or easygoing. When Reuben did not wake up early one morning, Isaac did not take him to day camp that afternoon. He decided that Reuben could stay at the house with nothing to do, and the boy seemed to go along with this.

Isaac: Should I allow him to do whatever he pleases?

Therapist: At the beginning of the summer, you said it would be a miracle if he went to camp. You never dreamed he could do it. Even the camp said that although he became stressed, he was successful and had a good month. A part of you is very pleased and proud, but I suspect another part of you is frightened and maybe threatened by the fact that he was able to go and is growing up. By demanding more of him now, you may be stretching him to the limit. It's as if you are punishing him for separating. I'm not saying this is intentional or that you're a bad parent. I think it's that you are frightened of the changes. Last year, you gave him the message that it was permissible to separate when you made him go to school every day. As much as you want him to do well, there may be a feeling of loss— that he no longer needs you in the same way.

Isaac later described this session as a turning point in terms of lessening the destructive forces within. In our discussion, I initially went too far in emphasizing how destructive it was for Reuben to remain home without anything to do. Isaac did not accept my statements and we nearly argued. It rang true for him when I remarked that he was punishing Reuben for his success because he was threatened by loss. He astutely remarked it was not only that he felt a sense of loss but that he attacked his own success at helping Reuben to separate. The inner parental tyrant that attacked Isaac now directed its aggression against his son. Isaac realized that when Reuben became very resistant or stubborn, he was frightened and in need of empathy. Instead, Isaac either overindulged him by permitting him to remain at home or became angry and punitive.

For the coming year, Reuben was to start a new school and was expected to take the school bus. In the past, Isaac had always driven him to school, so Reuben was now resistant to the change. Isaac was able to acknowledge his vulnerability and fear, comfort him, but encourage him to go. He became increasingly aware of how his own parents had undermined him. On one occasion when he was pleased with himself, his son, and his family, he spoke to his mother on the phone and praised his son. His mother did not respond but instead asked, in a critical way, about problems she had known Reuben to have. He felt that she was saying, "Don't think you're so smart. If you're so smart, why does Reuben have so many problems? You'd better not be too quick to forget that."

Thus internal persecutor objects attacked the vulnerable libidinal self's need for good object experience that could serve autonomy. The attacks of the persecutory objects brought out the regressed ego's need to retreat and withdraw. The good object could only be protected from bad objects by maintaining it in a highly idealized position personified as God.

Example 2

Basing her views on Rosenfeld's concept of destructive narcissism, Betty Joseph (1982) described patients with a malignant type of self-destructiveness, which she aptly described as an addiction to near-death. This is not a drive toward a nirvanalike peaceful state but rather a pull toward helplessness, despair, and activities that are extremely self-destructive, both mentally and physically. These patients may engage in overworking, poor sleeping habits, overeating, excessive drinking, and destructive relationships. They are prone to experiencing a negative therapeutic reaction, but this is only part of a much broader and insidious pull toward self-destruction. Whereas Betty Joseph emphasized the death instinct, I believe that there is a tie to an early destructive relationship with no internal ideal object to neutralize its effects.

Mary was an adult patient in her mid-thirties who came to the clinic because she was depressed and suicidal. She was despondent because she had been in a relationship with a married man for several years and he had refused to leave his physically ill wife. The man was an executive and Mary was the manager at his office. In the consultation interview, she said that she planned to kill herself if he did not leave his wife. Over the next couple of weeks, Mary put her plan into action. She took nearly lethal doses of barbiturates mixed with alcohol, saying that she was flirting with death. I met with Mary and her lover together. He said he was consumed by guilt over Mary's depression but could not leave his wife because she was physically ill. He said that he had ruined the lives of both his wife and Mary and was entirely at fault. Mary said she felt terrible that she had placed him in this position and would kill herself to end their misery. He said he would feel worse knowing she had killed herself. She replied that he'd be unhappy for only a short while, then would feel better.

I felt that Mary came to the clinic so that a therapist could convince her lover how disturbed and serious she was so that he would leave his wife. She showed no conscious wish to stop playing this Russian roulette with her life or to receive help for her depression. I felt that, since she continued to come to the clinic, she wanted help on some level. Therefore, I continued to see her.

In subsequent sessions, I attempted to get Mary in touch with her anger toward her lover for not leaving his wife. I explained that she turned anger at him against herself. These interpretations had little effect. She understood my remarks intellectually but had no wish to live without him.

Mary described a life history filled with severe familial emotional neglect. In her adolescence she had made a serious suicide attempt. Before meeting her married lover, she had been severely depressed and had felt that there was little to live for. Her lover, who was an older man, had treated her as if she were special, and for the first time she felt that there was something to live for.

At first, she was satisfied with seeing him occasionally. Over time, however, she became depressed again. She believed it was because he would not give himself completely over to her. Yet some part of her wondered if the initial euphoria over the relationship was wearing off and she was returning to her original depressed state. Maybe she needed more of him to counteract the return of her depression because the comforting effects of the relationship were wearing off. In lucid moments, she could think all of this through, but then the depression came over her and she could only think that she would not be able to live without her lover. When she became angry at him, she did not feel better because then the only comfort in her life—that she was in some way accepted by this valued and loved man—was lost. She was merely an unworthy person rejected by an uncaring lover.

During the weeks I was seeing Mary on a daily basis, I was arranging for her to meet with the clinic's psychiatrists. She did not wish to go to a psychiatric hospital and knew what to say to them to avoid being committed. Nevertheless, the psychiatrists were of the opinion that she needed to be hospitalized, and we attempted to convince her to sign herself in.

Mary usually kept her daily appointments at the clinic, but occasionally, if she took too many pills the night before, she neither came nor called. During the several weeks that I met with her, it was like being on an emotional roller coaster. There was much suspense about whether she would make it through the day, whether we could get her to go to a hospital. When I met with her, I was either greatly relieved that she seemed slightly better or frightened that she seemed to be losing all control. Mary reported driving her car into a pole. She described going into dangerous neighborhoods carrying a knife and blindly walking the streets, hoping someone would start with her so that she could end her misery "one way or another." One day she came to the session so drugged that she could not stay awake or talk. I called the emergency number and she was hospitalized in a psychiatric ward for one week. I attempted to convince her to stay longer, but she signed herself out.

As soon as Mary was discharged, she resumed playing Russian roulette by mixing pills and alcohol. I convinced her to visit a psychiatric hospital with me, not to sign herself in but to see what it was like. I explained that unlike the hospital she had just left, the one I wanted her to see kept patients longer and had more means to help. She agreed to visit but did not keep the appointment. During this period, her pull toward death became more intense. She said she thought of killing her lover, herself, and me with a rifle. She kept a rifle under her bed, and she sometimes took it to the country and fired it to let off steam. I was frightened by her remarks but thought that she was trying to drive me away from helping her. I told her this and also that she was terrified of going into a hospital and separating from the few persons to whom she was attached. Therefore, she had the idea of all of us going together.

Shortly thereafter, Mary called to say she had written a suicide note. She read it to me over the phone and said goodbye. I told her that she was again rejecting the help I could provide, that her mistrust was understandable given all of the times she had been disappointed by people. I reminded her how she had said that I was doing all that I could to help, but now she was treating my help as worthless, which implied that she, the recipient of my help, was worthless.

I had a sense that her call was meant not only to inform me of the suicide note but to make contact. Several days later we visited the psychiatric hospital together. We met with the admissions psychiatrist and toured the wards and spacious grounds. Mary was comfortable and said that the hospital was more attractive than she had expected. She and the staff psychiatrist agreed on an admissions date for the following week.

I saw Mary every day. It was agreed that on the day of the admission she and her lover would come to the clinic and we would all go to the hospital. She telephoned the night before we were to go and said she wanted me to know that she would come. The call was unusual. She had never before telephoned to say she was or was not coming.

Mary did not show up the next morning. I thought that the phone call had been a signal. Calling to assure me she would come meant that if she did not, something was wrong. I called her lover at his job. She was supposed to have met him at work and they were to come to the clinic together. He said that she had never arrived and that she must not have been serious about going to the hospital. I insisted that he meet me at her apartment since he had a key. When we arrived there, Mary was unconscious. We tried to wake her but without success. Her body was deadweight, like a carcass, but she was breathing. The ambulance arrived and rushed her to the hospital. She was in a coma from a drug overdose, and it was several days before she came out of it. She left the medical hospital for direct admission to the psychiatric hospital. After being there a few days, she wanted to sign herself out. A hearing was held and she was committed. One of the psychiatrists said that she was the most suicidal patient he had ever seen on the ward. Mary called me after she had been there several weeks to say she was feeling less suicidal.

Guntrip (1969) stated that the regressed ego is characterized by the vegetative passivity of the intrauterine state. However, the regressed ego can display great energy and urgent activity in its retreat from life. Mary reached a state of oblivion through her drugged states. Her wish to die was not only a turning of rage against herself but a last-ditch effort to escape from a life that she

found too painful and difficult to cope with. Mary was retreating to
a regressed, withdrawn state well before meeting her lover. At first,
he represented the ideal object who would rescue her from an
objectless state. In her desperate effort to possess him, he was
transformed into an exciting and rejecting object. She was caught
between her fear of internal bad objects and her terror of objectlessness. For Mary, there was hardly any sense of an internal good
object to warm, comfort, and protect her from the regressed ego.

In the short time I worked with her, the question was whether
she would enter the hospital and allow for the possibility of a
therapeutic regressive experience or whether the regressed ego
could only escape through suicide. I endeavored to become enough
of a holding object to help her choose the hospital. A major dilemma
was that, for Mary, going into the hospital evoked severe separation anxiety, which reflected the terror of the regressed ego losing
all objects in its withdrawn state.

At the time I encountered this patient, I was not very experienced in practicing psychotherapy. Looking back, I wonder
whether my intense involvement in helping her go into a hospital
may have added to her separation anxiety and made it more difficult
for her to go. On the other hand, my involvement enabled her to
have some inner sense of the possibility of good object relations and
may have contributed to her signaling me for help. Searles (1965)
remarked that when the patient and therapist establish a therapeutic
relationship, the communication becomes increasingly nonverbal
and unconscious. I understood Mary's call the night before the
planned admission to be a promise that she would come. That
meant that if she did not come it wasn't that she simply stayed away,
but that she was in trouble. The phone call implied that she trusted
me to trust her not to consciously break her promise and to recognize her call for help. While the phone call was a clear communication, the actual overdose may have been an enactment, not a
communication. Mary enacted her equation of going to the hospital
with death and the ultimate loss of all objects. Another part of her
mind was aware of the impending unconscious enactment and
called for help. There was a part of her that wanted to remain alive
and in contact with objects from the beginning, and it is this part of
her that brought her to the clinic for help in the first place.

PART THREE

INTERPRETING AND HOLDING IN THE THERAPEUTIC PROCESS

9

THE TREATMENT OF
A BORDERLINE
PATIENT

The following case vignette describes seven years of treatment of a borderline patient. In this case it was necessary for the therapist to shore up separateness through the paternal function of interpretation. Only after this was done could the patient be offered a holding relationship, which could provide an opportunity for the formation of new self-structure. The following treatment first focused on the depressive conflict and only later analyzed underlying schizoid splitting of the personality. The patient was seen in weekly sessions, throughout the course of treatment.

Irene was a middle-aged patient who worked as a foster care counselor. She presented difficulties relating to her adolescent daughter and male lover. She complained that her lover was unavailable, saw other women, and was self-preoccupied. She said that her daughter did not study for school, spent all of her time out with friends, and did not obey. Irene felt helpless and out of control in both relationships. Irene was a middle child with a brother a year older than she and another brother two years younger.

HISTORY

Irene grew up in a middle-class family. When she was an infant, her mother had focused little attention on her. Her mother was in her late teens when she gave birth and had not been prepared to raise a child. In the first year of Irene's life, her mother became physically ill and neglected her to the point that she sometimes went hungry. The maternal grandmother came to live with them, providing Irene with whatever care she received. As a child, Irene tried to be helpful by cleaning, shopping, and readily doing chores. She was hard-working, did well academically, and was obedient at home. She once asked her mother why she was not praised for her achievement. Her mother said, "You are just that way. I never expect anything less from you."

Irene's father was an alcoholic and a gambler. He was away most of the time, and the parents divorced when Irene was 6. The grandmother took care of Irene. She loved to feed her and hold her and show off how pretty she was. Irene was heartbroken when her grandmother had to be hospitalized. Irene was 6 years old. The grandmother was diagnosed as paranoid-schizophrenic and was repeatedly hospitalized for the rest of her life. Irene felt that she had irretrievably lost her at age 6.

Irene emphasized that her mother was never a cruel or abusive person. She rarely hit or scolded Irene. She was well liked, sociable, and friendly. Irene was angry at her mother for her neglect as a young child but was ambivalent about the treatment she received as an adolescent. Her mother treated Irene more like a friend than a daughter, telling Irene to call her by her first name, trusting her to stay out as late as she wished, to do whatever she wanted, and to date whomever she pleased. Her mother was very open about discussing birth control and sexuality and was understanding and available if Irene had trouble with boyfriends. Irene's friends loved to talk to her mother and envied Irene for having such a with-it parent. Irene enjoyed the increased contact and interest of her mother, yet resented her for the childhood neglect. On the one hand, she felt that her mother liked her but on the other hand she wondered how much of her mother's libertarian attitude reflected a lack of genuine concern.

Irene's older brother was her mother's favorite. He did poorly in school but was athletic and popular with his peers. Irene was angry that if he received a C, her mother reacted as if he had just won a gold medal. She said that he must be a genius because he received the grade without even trying. Irene sometimes felt so angry that she wished him dead. She also wished that he would fail so that her mother would learn that he was unworthy of her love. The brother grew up to be a corporate executive. Irene complained that he never invited her to visit or to have dinner with him. She described her younger brother as lazy, manipulative, and considerably less successful than her older sibling. Irene said he took after their father, becoming an alcoholic and a gambler and later marrying, having children, and deserting his family.

Irene graduated college after having earned good grades. She married a man remarkably similar to her father. He drank and gambled and they divorced after having a daughter. Irene underwent considerable emotional turmoil raising a young child single-handedly. She was subject to severe anxiety and depression and became addicted to Valium. She saw a therapist for a couple of years who helped her to get off Valium and to function on a job. She said that the therapist had provided her with important help in functioning and controlling her distressed feelings and impulses, but that there had not been any significant change in her overall personality. She continued to feel helpless, unworthy, dependent, and enraged, although she no longer let her feelings get altogether out of control. She discontinued treatment when her therapist retired.

INTERPRETATIONS TO ESTABLISH SEPARATENESS

In the beginning of treatment, Irene focused on her relationship with her 16-year-old daughter, Alice. Irene never allowed Alice to cry as a baby. Whenever Alice was unhappy, Irene fed her. Shortly thereafter, Alice began to reject food. She never became fully anorexic but grew up to be a fussy eater. Food remained a source of conflict between mother and daughter. Irene angrily complained that Alice would not eat after she had gone through considerable

trouble to prepare dinner. I empathized with Irene about the difficulties in parenting an adolescent but pointed to the extent of her
rage as being out of proportion to the situation. I remarked on the
hurt and feelings of rejection underlying her rage.

Irene always put Alice first. Although she earned enough
money to afford a middle-class lifestyle, finances remained difficult.
If there was money for only one dress, it went to Alice. Irene took
great pride in how pretty her daughter was. Alice increasingly was
more interested in her appearance, her friends, and good times than
she was in her studies, her family, or her responsibilities. Irene and
she constantly fought over the girl's lack of responsibility. The
fights often became violent. Irene sometimes threw her daughter
out of the house or refused to pay for appropriate items. Although
Alice did not excel in school, she also did not fail. However, when
Irene was in a rage, she forgot about any of Alice's positive characteristics. If I pointed this out, Irene turned her rage on me. She said,
"So you think it's fine for her to fail" or "What should I do, buy her
whatever she wants?" or "Should I just allow her to come home
whenever she wishes?" I interpreted splitting by pointing out that
when Alice disappointed the mother, Irene became disappointed in
herself as a mother and disappointed in Alice. There was no separation. Alice's failure meant that Irene failed as a mother. Furthermore, Irene had lost all perspective, seeing Alice or what she did
never as half bad but as all bad, and seeing herself in the same way.
I said, "You see yourself and Alice as the worst mother–daughter
pair of all time." These interpretations had a calming effect on Irene,
but I had to say them repeatedly, strongly, and firmly to cut
through her depression and rage.

I acknowledged that there was a realistic side to her complaints
but that they did not merely reflect her concerns about Alice. I said,
"Alice's overinvolvement in her appearance and social life, her lack
of responsibility, could apply to the descriptions you've given of
your own mother's behavior. The way you have sacrificed yourself
for Alice is identical to how you described sacrificing yourself for
your mother. As a child you cleaned, did chores, and shopped so
that she would come to appreciate you, take care of you, and not
abandon you. When you are angry that you have done so much for
Alice and get nothing in return, you are reliving the anger you felt
toward your mother for not taking proper care of you."

Irene became aware that she believed her daughter took after her own mother. I interpreted that she attempted to create her own mother out of the daughter because she still needed her mother. The daughter's growing up and separating was unconsciously equated with the mother's emotional abandonment of her. Irene said that during her childhood, she rarely felt angry at her mother. I stated that the anger was probably repressed and that what she now felt toward Alice was likely that repressed anger toward her mother.

Irene's complaints about her boyfriend were along similar lines. She sacrificed her time, money, and love, yet he remained narcissistic and unavailable. She felt that he gave his attention to other, less deserving persons while putting her last. I compared this situation to that of her mother's giving attention to her less deserving older brother. Interpretations regarding both the daughter and boyfriend provided the paternal function of helping her to separate from the preoedipal mother. Irene was often angry at me for providing interpretations instead of simply understanding how she felt. Some of the rage could be attributed to the fact that I was attempting to effect separation from the early symbiotic union. This period covered nearly the first five years of treatment. I also provided a maternal holding function by remaining available for phone calls or extra needed appointments. I doubt that she could have tolerated the interpretive work without the coinciding emotional availability. Wright (1991d) finds that the therapist sometimes must provide a securely held space of separateness before the patient can tolerate playing in a held, potential space without resorting to merger or the denial of separateness. During this period, Irene broke up with her boyfriend and her daughter moved out of state. Irene had to become accustomed to living independently. She made new friends and became involved in new recreational and social activities. As she became more autonomous, I provided more of a holding relationship.

PLAYING WITH IDEAS AND POSSIBILITIES

Winnicott recommended that therapy should at times come as close as possible to approximating play. In the treatment of an adult patient, he (1972) described how the patient expressed an inclination to play in an intellectual way, by playing with ideas about himself or others. This experience permitted the patient to free himself from the dominance of rigid internalized object relations units and reified defenses. Irene began to play with ideas of what motivates herself and others. She attempted to decide whether her daughter was distant and quarrelsome because Irene was a bad mother or whether she had her own motives and interests. Irene realized that her daughter had her own conflicts around autonomy and became aware of how her own insecurities sometimes contributed to the daughter's need to fight her off. She now actively explored whether her impulses to make demands upon or to reject others were warranted by realistic consideration of the situation or whether she was reacting to internal fears of closeness or separateness. I rarely provided direct answers but rather stimulated her to think of different possibilities. There was a radical change in her descriptions of relationships. She now was often thoughtful, intellectually playful, and relatively calm.

MANIC DEFENSE OR PRACTICING AUTONOMY?

There continued to be the quality of a manic defense about Irene's efforts to be more on her own. She developed a circle of friends and filled every spare moment of her time with a planned activity. Her time was so booked up that if someone called her unexpectedly, she never had any free time for the foreseeable future. She did not differentiate among her circle of friends, but instead saw everyone as interchangeable. They were people to do things with. If someone disappointed her, she did not mind so long as she had someone to replace that person. At times she felt so busy and exhausted that she was near collapse. However, it was better to be busy and active, she said, than to feel depressed and abandoned.

Winnicott (1971a) described how doing is authentic if it is based on a firm foundation of being. The desperate compulsivity of Irene's doing suggested an underlying ego weakness. I could have interpreted that her compulsive activity was an effort to escape from feelings of abandonment and depression or gone even deeper to say that her desperate doing endeavored to fill a void or lack in her state of being. Although both interpretations would have been accurate, it would have been a mistake to make either. They missed the crucial point that it was an indication of greater ego strength on her part that she was actively bringing herself to socialize with people and to avoid situations in which she undoubtedly would have felt depressed or lacking. Therefore, I continually remarked that going to movies, dining out, and socializing with friends were all indications of greater autonomy.

Melanie Klein (1935) defined the manic defense as a phantasy of omnipotent control over internal objects giving rise to a state of elation of triumph over loss. Irene's effort to relate to objects as interchangeable and not important in their own right suggested a manic defense. However, her earlier attempts to control her daughter and boyfriend were examples of an extensive use of that defense. Therefore, Irene was now employing the manic defense less extensively. Mahler (1975) suggested that elation accompanies the practicing subphase of separation-individuation through which the toddler feels on top of the world. Objects interchangeably serve refueling so that the child may explore the surrounding world. In this case, Irene reverted to practicing subphase experience to effect separation from the object. Mahler stated that the practicing may be accompanied by elation because of the flight from engulfment but did not believe that this behavior was intentional, rather that its effects could become intentional. Irene's original efforts to effect separation were accompanied by the elation felt by the flight from fusion. In all likelihood, there was an unconscious phantasy of omnipotent control over the object—being able to escape from it but return to it at will—that made the initial separation tolerable. Irene's overactivity was less destructive than her former controlling behavior and served her efforts to practice autonomy. I therefore provided support with little interpretation.

THE REVELATION OF A HIDDEN EATING DISORDER

Irene continued on her frantic merry-go-round of activity for a couple of years until she started to complain of a lack of intimacy in

her life. After breaking up with her boyfriend, she had first avoided
dating, fearing losing her autonomy or being exploited. She now
started to see men. She complained that they were demanding and
impatient and that they in turn accused her of being selfish and
manipulative. She dismissed most of their complaints as unjustified,
but she was struck by something one man had said. He had accused
her of using him for a meal ticket. She said that there was truth to his
remark. She was a fussy eater and panicked over the possibility of
not finding the food she preferred. She liked to dine in fine restaurants, but the panic that she felt at not getting a good dinner was far
beyond rational bounds. She planned the entire day around eating.
If a man asked her out, she had to know beforehand where and
when they would eat. She was expert at getting her way without
being conspicuous.

I first raised some questions as to the nature and severity of the
problem. I stated that the wish to dine in a fine restaurant reflected
a capacity to enjoy herself. It was not a problem in itself. I wondered
whether her definition of it as a problem could be reflective of a
need to discourage or criticize herself for treating herself well or
enjoying herself. She said that the issue went well beyond enjoying
a good dinner. Her refrigerator was always stuffed beyond any
sensible degree. She panicked at the idea of being hungry. The mere
thought of being in a situation where she could be hungry but not
get food brought on a panic attack. She added that it was not easy to
detect her compulsive behavior around food because she was not
overweight, but she often ate compulsively when upset. She sometimes overate to the point of being nauseous but did not vomit. She
binged when she felt abandoned or rejected.

It was during this discussion that Irene recalled that her grandmother had informed her that her mother had been physically ill
during Irene's infancy and the fact that Irene sometimes went
hungry. I remarked that the relationship between the infant and
mother is experienced through the medium of food and that the
baby comes to associate being fed with being loved. Being deprived
of food thus came to be associated with being unloved and abandoned. I said that hunger threatened her with annihilation as an
infant. Chronic hunger is felt by a baby as the threat and pain of
annihilation and the feeling of being unloved and abandoned.

Irene's panic attacks over food were a reliving of the early threat of abandonment and annihilation. She attempted to ward off these feelings by always having access to food.

Irene responded to this interpretation by remembering how she had always fed her infant daughter, even when she was not hungry. She said, "I must have fed her as I wished to be fed as an infant. Alice came to be a fussy bad eater, like my own mother. It's strange how history repeats itself. My grandmother tried to feed my mother, just as I always tried to feed Alice. I felt rejected when Alice didn't want my food. Maybe my grandmother felt rejected when my mother didn't want her food." Thus Irene was the ghost of her grandmother and Alice the ghost of Irene's mother.

THE ANALYSIS OF DEPRESSIVE CONFLICT

As Irene became aware of her abandonment anxiety, the death of her mother became the treatment focus. The mother had been terminally ill for a year when Irene was an adult, and it had fallen to Irene to take care of her. For the first time she confronted her mother for neglecting her as a child. Her mother had reacted with surprise and denied her maltreatment of Irene. Irene became so angry that she literally spit in her eye. After her mother died, Irene felt pained and guilty. In fact, the pain itself was physical and was manifested in her chest.

I remarked that her lifelong ambivalent feelings toward her mother contributed to the sense that Irene had injured or destroyed her. The phantasy of angry wishes destroying the mother was reinforced by her behavior directly preceding her mother's death. In addressing a patient's rage toward a significant object, it is important to support any positive feelings that exist so that the patient is not threatened with anxiety over losing even the good aspects of the object. This point is especially important for those patients who have a weak or tenuous internal positive object image. I emphasized that Irene's anger toward her mother was due to the fact that she also loved and needed her and that her impending loss therefore frightened and angered her.

Irene experienced similar ambivalence toward her older brother, who had recently lost his job and all of his money. When she had begun treatment, she complained that he was wealthy but never helped her. She also resented him because he was her mother's favorite. The tables were now turned as he came to her for help.

When Irene spoke of the pain she felt at her mother's death, she touched her chest, emphasizing its physical nature.

> *Therapist*: You feel pained at the pain that you feel you caused your mother when she was dying. You keep your mother with you by feeling her pain in your chest. There is the feeling of having caused her pain, and now there is the retaliation of that pain in your chest.
>
> *Irene*: It is like someone stabbing me in the chest with a knife.
>
> *Therapist*: The mother you phantasized injuring now persecutes you with the stabbing pains in the chest. This is the pain of your guilty feelings.

Irene again raised the issue of guilt over her brother. I interpreted that when she was little she may have felt that the brother had everything because he had their mother. She secretly may have hoped that he would someday lose everything. She recalled wishing that her brother and mother would die. I said now that her mother was dead and her brother had lost all of his money, she was feeling that her childhood wishes had been fulfilled. Thus she felt guilty and was punishing herself and keeping her mother with her through the pain. She wondered if it was common to feel a lost person inside oneself. I said, "The feelings about the lost person are taken inside as if they *are* the lost person." Irene recalled her tendency to binge on food after feeling abandoned. She now understood that this was her way of incorporating the lost object.

THE ATTRACTION TO THE UNPREDICTABILITY OF THE OBJECT

Shortly thereafter, Irene began to see a new man. He took her to fine restaurants, said she was the most special person he ever knew, and was ready to do whatever she wished. She was taken by his attentiveness, feeling better about him than anyone else she had dated. Problems soon emerged, however. When she would ready herself to go to work, after having spent the night with him, he would continually interrupt, forcing her to be late. If he had a day off, he would try to convince her to take the day off also. If she insisted on going to work, he would act as if she had rejected him. If she planned to meet a friend, he would become especially interested in convincing her to change her plans and to see him. He increasingly demanded that she be available when he wished, but he refused to be pinned down if she wished to see him. He would never commit himself as to when he would call or see her. I remarked that by his behavior he repeatedly excited her interest and then rejected her. She acknowledged feeling more excited by him than by the other men she had known. I explored what excited her about him. As she described his characteristics and behavior, she continually returned to his unpredictability. She never knew whether he would call or what mood he would be in. It was the unpredictability itself that excited her.

THE REVELATION OF THE IDEAL OBJECT

Irene became interested in what hooked her on this man. She thought that the way he treated her as special originally was an important factor. I asked her who in her childhood treated her as special. She said that her parents never did, but then thought of her grandmother. Her grandmother loved to feed her. She also gave Irene whatever she wanted and told her she would grow up to be Miss America. Irene realized that she expected the man to feed her, give her whatever she wanted, and love her unconditionally, recreating the ideal love of her grandmother.

THE INTERPRETATION OF PRIMITIVE SPLITTING

I reminded Irene of her first year of life. Her mother was ill and she went hungry. Her grandmother probably saved her emotional and physical life. Her grandmother fed her and loved her and thereby drove away the early threat of annihilation and abandonment. In terms of endopsychic structure, Irene projected the ideal object onto the nurturing grandmother, which allowed her to repress and split off the earlier exciting abandoning mother. Her grandmother eventually disappointed her by going away to the psychiatric hospital.

THE EMERGENCE OF EARLY DEPRIVATION IN THE TRANSFERENCE

Irene said that she sometimes felt starved after our sessions and binged on food. I interpreted that she attempted to avoid feeling loss, abandonment, and emptiness. The food represented the nurturing grandmother, and she used it to avoid feeling the deprivation and rage toward me that she had felt toward her mother. She wondered if her grandmother could have been so perfect. After all, she had been diagnosed as paranoid-schizophrenic. Irene gradually recalled memories in which her grandmother was sometimes unpredictable and unreliable. Similarly, her current boyfriend originally treated her as special but then became increasingly erratic and rejecting. She imagined that this followed the pattern of her experience with her grandmother

At this point, Irene began to risk experiencing emptiness and separateness. I now interpreted that the way she filled all of her time was an effort to avoid the original emptiness or absence of the mother. Such behavior does not allow for anything spontaneous or novel to occur. She tried to stop filling herself with food and activities and allowed for some unplanned time. She became extremely anxious but could not understand why. I said that emptiness revived the early longing for the mother. Intellectually, she was aware that the mother was dead and would not return. Thus she was not likely to long for the person of the mother. However, the longings for the mother remained alive in the transference, since as her therapist I was the person she came to for help. I stated that she feared feeling the sense of loss when she was separated from me between sessions.

Irene broke up with the boyfriend who mistreated her. While going with him she had felt that it was her fault that he rejected her.

She always wondered if she could do anything different to change him. She continually tried to change herself to change him. She said, "I feel it must somehow be my fault. I must be doing something wrong. It must be my hairstyle, my makeup, maybe my behavior. Maybe I'm too available. Maybe I'm not available enough. I drive myself crazy. It must be my fault, I must be doing something, that I must in some way not be worthwhile if he treats me this way." I interpreted that as a child, when a parent treated her badly, she must have felt it was because she was not worthwhile, that there must be something wrong with her. I pointed out that a child develops a positive or negative self-image based on how the parent feels about the child. When the object mistreats the child, the child feels the object to be bad for mistreating her but feels that she is mistreated because she is at fault, unworthy. Thus the object's badness is attributed to the self. Fairbairn (1943) believed that the child internalized the badness of the object to protect the needed relationship with the object. Sartre (1943) provide an additional explanation—that the self forms in response to the object.

As Irene no longer attempted to always close the gap of separation, she experienced longing and deprivation in the transference. The pain of the interval between sessions and her longing for the next appointment were a reliving of the early deprivation and waiting for the next feeding. She said, "I literally feel that I can't live till the next session. I am panicked something will happen to you or me. Here I am an adult, a professional self-supporting person who raised a child, yet I feel so infantile and helpless—dying for the next session." I explained that as a baby between feedings, she must have been terrified of annihilation. When she spoke about dying to see me, the pain she had felt waiting until her next feeding must have been comparable to dying. I said her terror that the session would never come related to the fact that as an infant she did not have a basic sense of security to believe that her mother cared enough to return. It was the sense that I, like her mother, did not really care and would forget her because she was not worthwhile. This made the absences so painful and terrifying. As Irene gradually came to tolerate states of emptiness and separateness, she began to experience her authentic wishes and desires and to become less terrified of abandonment.

10

A RETURN TO THE CASE OF ANNA O.

The first case history to be recorded in psychoanalysis is that of Anna O. She was treated by Joseph Breuer, and her case was later discussed and written up by Breuer and Freud. They credited her for contributing to the discovery of the "talking cure." In the latter part of her life Anna O. became one of the most important social workers in Germany. According to Lucy Freeman (1972), her achievements are comparable to those of Jane Addams in the United States. Anna O., whose real name was Bertha Pappenheim, is now known and honored for her contributions to psychoanalysis and social work. Interestingly, the professions of psychoanalysis and social work became related in the United States in providing help for environmentally disadvantaged clients of social service agencies. Psychoanalysis provided social work with a theoretical model of the personality, while social work influenced analyis in recognizing the importance of supportive management and a holding environment (Winnicott 1963). Social workers such as Annette Garret, Florence Hollis, and Gordon Hamilton included supportive management in the principles of social work practice, and Bertha Pappenheim was among the first to provide a holding environment for socially disadvantaged children and young women. Object relations analysts such as Fairbairn, Guntrip, and Winnicott provided a scientific developmental understanding of the infant–mother relationship as a basis for holding and supportive management principles of therapy.

Anna O. suffered from a condition diagnosed as hysteria, which originally was thought to be a disease that affected women exclusively. The condition (from the Greek *hystera*, meaning uterus or womb), was once believed to be caused by a wandering womb, and patients were typically labeled as malingerers. The idea that hysteria may have psychological origins was introduced in the mid-1880s by the renowned French clinician Jean Martin Charcot and by Sigmund Freud in Vienna. Freud was ridiculed for believing that men could also suffer from the condition and that patients were not malingerers but exhibited a disorder of the mind.

Joseph Breuer treated Anna O. from December 1880 to June 1882. Breuer at the time was a reputable and successful doctor whose patients included Brahms and Bruckner. Freud was a 25-year-old neurology student when Breuer described the case to him. He was fascinated and intrigued by Anna O. and persuaded Breuer to include the case in their collaboration on *Studies on Hysteria*.

CASE NARRATIVE

Anna O. was born in 1859 into a wealthy Orthodox Jewish family in Vienna. She was proud of her family tree, which included the poet Heinrich Heine, and kept a genealogy tacked on her wall until her death. She had a younger brother, Wilhelm, and two older sisters, who died. Anna O.'s upbringing and education were typical of a girl of her social class—she was fluent in English, Italian, and French and well versed in literature and art. Breuer (Freud and Breuer 1895) described her as a remarkably intelligent, attractive, and sociable young woman with a keen intuition, and was much interested in helping the poor and infirm. However, she lived an extremely monotonous existence in a rigid, puritanical family and was subject to excessive fantasizing and extreme mood shifts. Breuer remarked that she appeared present when spoken to so that no one was aware that she was living in the fairy tales of her imagination.

Anna O. first suffered hysteria in 1880 when her father became ill and bedridden from a peripleuritic abscess. She nursed him, sitting by his bedside for five months until she herself collapsed. Her symptoms included paralysis of three limbs, severe headaches, disturbed vision, an inability to eat, a severe cough, shifts from intense excitement to exhaustion, and complaints that the walls of her room were collapsing.

During this period she experienced a radical splitting off of ego states. She sometimes recognized her environment, went for walks, and was lucid and sensible. She described this state as an expression of her "good self," which Breuer (Freud and Breuer 1895) thought of as "melancholy and anxious, but relatively normal" (p. 76). During the alternating state, which she described as her "naughty self," she would throw pillows, accuse people of tormenting her, and hallucinate. She experienced a gap in her thinking and a loss of time, especially in reaction to someone entering or leaving the room or starting to move about. These states of consciousness alternated rapidly and became increasingly distinct. During her father's illness she sometimes hallucinated snakes and death's-heads and would babble. She was in a semi-sleeping state through most afternoons, then would awaken and feel tormented an hour or so after sunset. She gradually lost the power of speech and writing and for two weeks became entirely silent. Breuer recognized that her silence occurred after he had said something that may have been offensive. He encouraged her to talk about it, and the inhibition disappeared. Her paralysis also began to recede. She only spoke English but understood her native language of German when others spoke.

Anna O.'s father died April 5, 1881, when she was 22. She had seen him only rarely during the last stage of his illness and suffered her worst setback immediately following his death. She initially reacted with violent excitement, then withdrew into a stupor for two days. She emerged in a semi-withdrawn state and was quieter, although her arm and legs remained paralyzed. There was also some restriction in her field of vision. For instance, she saw only one flower at a time when presented with a bouquet, although flowers had ordinarily given her considerable pleasure. She barely recognized people and had "to do laborious recognizing work and had to say to herself this person's nose is such-and-such, his face is such-and-such, he must be so-and-so" (pp. 78–79). She perceived people to look like wax figures and she could recognize those she was ordinarily pleased to see for only a short while. Breuer had been visiting her once a day (an extraordinary amount of time for a physician to devote to a patient during that period) and she had grown attached to him. He was the only one she consistently recognized, and she remained lively and in contact while he spoke to her. On one visit he brought along another physician. She completely ignored the new doctor, responding only to Breuer's questions. The other physician rather insensitively tried to break through to her by blowing smoke in her face. She suddenly hallu-cinated a stranger before her, rushed to the door for the key, and collapsed. When Breuer had to leave Vienna for several days, Anna refused food and hallucinated terrifying death's-heads and skele-tons during his absence.

Breuer's treatment method followed a typical pattern. Anna was in a semi-hallucinatory state all day, and Breuer would hypno-tize her after sunset. Sometimes she was already in an autohypnotic state when he arrived. She invented the term "clouds" to refer to the hypnotic state. After she narrated the hallucinations she had expe-rienced during the day, she would become calm and cheerful through the evening. She could work, draw, and write until bed-time. During the day, she was pursued by hallucinations, but at night she was lucid and clear-minded.

Her psychic condition worsened despite Breuer's efforts and the pleasant evenings. She had strong suicidal impulses and could no longer be allowed to live on the third floor for fear she would throw herself from a window. She was moved to a country house outside Vienna, where she stayed on the first floor. There were numerous suicide attempts involving smashed windows, but they were less serious in the new residence. For the next twelve months, Anna O. was in her worst, most desperate state. She slept during the day but would mutter to herself, suggesting a tormented state. At night, she slept for about an hour, then would awaken uttering words of distress. She was encouraged to continue talking and soon began to tell stories that were sad but charming in style, like fairy tales. The stories centered on a girl sitting anxiously by a sickbed.

The completion of a narrative resulted in her fully awakening in a calmed state.

Breuer could no longer visit Anna every day because the new residence was too far away, but when he did visit her in the evening he would sometimes find her in an autohypnotic state. He would then relieve her of "the whole stock of imaginative products which she had accumulated" (p. 83) since his last visit. This left her calm, cheerful, and agreeable. The next day, however, she would return to being moody and would resist talking. She came to see that giving utterance to her hallucinations helped her to feel calm and more energetic. Nevertheless, Breuer had to plead and cajole her, sometimes repeating the way she typically introduced her stories to encourage her to talk. She aptly described the procedure she was engaged in with Breuer as the "talking cure," and jokingly referred to it as "chimney sweeping" (p. 83).

Anna's condition gradually improved. She allowed a nurse to feed her and her paralysis diminished. Breuer arranged to have his friend Dr. B. call on her when he himself could not visit. She became attached to a Newfoundland dog she was given. On one occasion, she had the energy to beat off her huge pet with a whip when it attacked a cat. She provided help for some sick and poor people, which lifted her spirits.

Breuer left for several weeks on holiday and returned to find Anna in a worsened condition. Although she had become devoted to Breuer's substitute, Dr. B., she would not carry on the "talking cure" with him. She was in a "wretched moral state, inert, unamenable, ill-tempered, even malicious" (p. 85). Breuer arranged for her to return to Vienna for a week and each evening had her narrate three to five stories. He stated that the pathogenic and exciting productions that had been accumulating over the several weeks of his absence now had a chance of being discharged. The "spontaneous productions" of her imagination persisted as a "psychic stimulus" until it could be released in narrative hypnosis.

In the fall of 1881 Anna returned to Vienna but to a different house. A year had passed since the onset of her condition. Breuer was astonished to discover that her consciousness was now divided. She lived part of the day in the present and part in the past exactly a year earlier. In one state she lived in the present period of the winter of 1881–1882, while in the other she lived in the winter of 1880–1881. In the new house, she hallucinated her old room and walked about it as if all of the furniture stood as it did in the former place and time. Breuer was confirmed in his view by a diary Anna O.'s mother had kept of 1881. For instance, one morning Anna felt angry at Breuer but had no idea why. He checked the diary and discovered that on the same day a year earlier he had annoyed her. On another occasion she could not discriminate colors and saw a brown dress she wore as blue. During the same period a year earlier, she had been working on a dressing gown for her father, which was the same material as her current dress but was blue instead of brown.

In the hypnotic work, Breuer had to focus not only on the contemporary "imaginative products" but also on the events and remembrances of 1881. In addition, he discovered that the psychical events of a third period, that of the incubation of the illness from July to December 1880, had an important role in the hysterical condition. Breuer believed that bringing memories to verbal release fully alleviated the symptoms. One of Anna's symptoms was an inability to drink water. This derived from witnessing an English-woman's dog drink water from a drinking glass. Although she was distressed, Anna had not protested. As she now recalled and described the event, the symptom disappeared entirely. Anna suffered from a chronic squint. She discovered and described how her squint went back to a night when her father had asked for the time and she could not reply because her eyes had been filled with tears.

Breuer visited Anna every morning to hypnotize her. He asked her to concentrate on a given symptom and recall and describe the occasions when it occurred. Anna recalled the symptom of not hearing when spoken to. She now recalled 108 separate occasions, listing persons, circumstances, and dates, when she did not hear. She concentrated on not comprehending when several people spoke together and recalled 27 separate incidents. She remembered 50 occasions when she was directly addressed when alone but could not hear. There were 37 instances when deafness was brought on by fright at a particular noise. As she talked through a symptom, it initially would emerge with greater intensity but then lessen.

Anna was determined to complete her treatment by June 7, the anniversary of the day that she had moved to the country. On the day she set for her recovery, she rearranged the furniture of her room to resemble her father's sickroom. She then reconstructed and relived the terrifying night that precipitated her illness. She had fallen asleep by her father's bedside with her right arm draped across the back of her chair. She had experienced a waking dream and saw a black snake coming toward her father to bite him. She tried to strike at the snake but was paralyzed. Her right arm had fallen asleep, and when she looked at it the fingers had turned into snakes with the nails as death's-heads. Through reliving this traumatic event and relieving her guilt over neglecting her father, the paralysis ended and the last of her symptoms disappeared.

After Breuer said goodbye to his "cured" patient, he was summoned back in an emergency. He found Anna undergoing a hysterical childbirth. She cried, "Dr. Breuer's child is coming!" Breuer sedated her and fled. He said that Anna had never discussed love or sexuality during the treatment. Over the next several years, Anna suffered relapses, was in and out of sanitoriums, became addicted to morphine and chloral, traveled, and slowly recovered her health. In the 1880s she and her mother went to Frankfurt, where she resumed her youthful interest in helping needy people.

History records two personifications of this patient. One is that of Anna O., the first recorded psychoanalytic patient who contributed to the discovery of the talking cure. The other is that of Bertha Pappenheim, who became one of the foremost social workers in Europe. She organized various German Jewish charities and educated, rehabilitated, and housed abandoned or transient Jewish children and young women. She utilized her personal fortune and influence to combat unjust social mores that left women and children with few rights. She struggled for the adoption of illegitimate children in a society that preferred to hide them in institutions. She also fought for the rights of women to divorce. A commemorative stamp issued by the West German government recognized her contributions to the organization of German Jewish charities.

In his analysis of Anna O., Breuer (Freud and Breuer 1895) emphasized the existence of two states of consciousness: a primary, relatively normal state and a secondary state, likened to a dream, constituted by a wealth of imaginary contents. He stated that the patient was lucid and well organized so long as the secondary state and the contents of the imagination did not intrude on the normal state. For the first time in his discussion, the phrase "in the unconscious" appeared. The contents of this secondary state were thought to be acting as a stimulus in the unconscious. Breuer said that the patient was "split into two personalities, one that was normal and the other insane" (p. 101). The "normal" side was described as "moral," the "insane" side as "bad." The unconscious stimulus was thought to intrude upon and disturb the normal side. Breuer believed that if the talking cure had not disposed of the stimulus, Anna would have become a hysteric of the "malicious type" characterized as "refractory, lazy, disagreeable and ill-natured" (p. 101).

Freud translated the "bad personality" of the hysteric into repressed instinctual impulses and the normal, moral personality into the ego and conscience (and later superego). Based on experience with hysterics, he developed his views on infantile sexuality and the sexual etiology of neurosis. He believed that Anna O.'s fantasized pregnancy reflected an erotic transference and that Breuer fled as a result of countertransference. Breuer disagreed with Freud's ideas of infantile sexuality and the sexual etiology of the neurosis. These differences in interpretation led to the rift in their relationship.

COMMENTARY

Breuer's view of dissociated subpersonalities and Freud's theory of repressed instinctual impulses are integrated in the contemporary object relations theory of split-off and repressed subselves that are inseparable from instinctual impulses.

Anna O.'s hysteric condition was brought on by the threatened loss of her father. The severity of her symptoms and the splitting of the ego suggest that the father served as an ideal internal object that was utilized to support the cohesion of a fragile self. The rage at the external object for the impending loss also threatened the positive introject with destruction (Klein 1940). Anna O.'s illness was precipitated by the attacks of the snakes on her ill father. When she looked at her paralyzed arm, she hallucinated that her fingers were snakes, her nails death's-heads. The snakes attacking her father reflected the phantasy of bad persecutory objects attacking the ideal object.

The loss of the external and internal ideal object left Anna at the mercy of the hallucinated bad objects. Guntrip (1969) described how the patient threatened by internal danger in the form of persecutory bad objects has no alternative but to take flight in a mental sense into a phantasized safety of a regressed, withdrawn ego state. Anna manifested a withdrawal from persecutory objects in her semi-sleeping state, and her inability to speak and write, which resulted in a period of utter silence. Following the death of her father, she withdrew further into a complete stupor, then emerged in a semi-withdrawn state. The extent of her withdrawal became apparent through Breuer's hypnotic efforts, which recalled incidents when she did not hear when spoken to, could not comprehend several persons talking together, and suffered deafness brought on by fright. All of these symptoms strongly suggest that the regressed ego had withdrawn from internal and external persecutory object relations. Guntrip (1969) said that regressed ego states were most likely the result of overwhelming impingement before the ego had the opportunity to form adequate protective boundaries. Anna O.'s deafness brought on by fright suggests extreme vulnerability to impingement.

Guntrip (1969) found that once a patient has retreated from outer reality to the fear-dictated state of the regressed ego, a conflict is set up between two opposing needs: the need to withdraw from intolerable reality and bad internal objects and the need to remain in touch with objects, even if bad, to avoid an objectless state. The flight into regression could then become a counterflight back into object relations. However, this return to object relations continues to result in persecution by bad objects and the need to return or remain in a withdrawn state. Anna O. was caught between this conflict of retreating to the regressed, withdrawn, but objectless state or returning to bad internal object relations. As Breuer pointed out, she was awakened from her semi-withdrawn states of consciousness by tormenting hallucinations and fantasies. Her "bad self" attempted to remain in contact by fighting with her inner bad objects. When the persecution became intolerable, she retreated to the passive, withdrawn state.

Anna's only hope was to establish a relationship to a good object to provide a buffer against persecution by bad objects and to reach the regressed, passive ego. Breuer clearly provided her with a supportive relationship. His descriptions of Anna's strengths, the extraordinary efforts he made, his devoted care, all demonstrated authentic concern for her wellbeing. Anna O. valued his support and, on occasion, emerged from her withdrawn, regressed states in response to his efforts. There was a time when Anna recognized and spoke to no one but Breuer. Nevertheless, despite his support, Breuer in some ways failed to provide her with a strong enough holding relationship. This failure resulted in her relapse. A closer look at how Breuer's support for Anna was lacking will prove relevant for understanding what constitutes a good holding relationship and how a therapist may partially fail in this endeavor even if he or she appears to be engaged in many overt procedures generally considered supportive.

THE I-YOU VERSUS I-IT RELATIONSHIP

Breuer remained unaware of the importance that the therapeutic relationship had for Anna. He reported leaving Anna in the care of a substitute physician, Dr. B., whom she already knew and liked, when he went away for a holiday. Breuer was surprised that she would not practice the talking cure with Dr. B. He returned to find her condition much worsened. The incident provided Breuer with the opportunity to question why Anna O. would engage in this activity only with him.

Breuer attributed all positive therapeutic results to his hypnotic technique. He believed that the patient suffered from innate stimuli that needed constant discharge through verbal utterance. Anna suffered a worsening of her condition when he went away because she lost the opportunity to release accumulated stimuli. For

Breuer, the therapeutic relationship was the medium for the talking cure. There was no understanding at the time that a fragile self achieved some cohesion through the relationship with an internal good object. When Breuer left, Anna relived the fragmentation of the self that had been caused by the loss of her father. The anger at Breuer as an external object for abandoning her by going away resulted in a rage reaction that threatened the internal, as well as external, good object relationship. Breuer provided Anna with a supportive external relationship but was unaware of her incapacity to internalize him as a good object during his absence.

Martin Buber (1958) distinguished two ways of relating in his philosophy of I–you and I–it relationships. He used the I–you situation to refer to two subjectivities primarily concerned with being, while the I–it relationship referred to doing in relation to a thinglike object. In the I–it relationship, the other is an object of analysis, the object of techniques. In the I–you relationship, there is primarily a sense of being together.

Breuer provided Anna with much support; however, the quality of the relationship was never I–you. Instead Breuer utilized techniques to alleviate her condition in the mode of the I doing to the it. Fairbairn (1941) stated that underlying the hysteric neurosis were the splitting of the ego and a schizoid psychic structure. Anna O. is a convincing example of Fairbairn's theory. She was in need of a holding relationship, the maternal function, to heal the early splits of the ego. The case report shows how a therapist may create a relationship more in the mode of I–it than I–you and therefore lacking as a holding relationship.

PSYCHIC REBIRTH AND THE OEDIPAL UNION

Anna O. announced the date of her cure, which culminated in the fantasy of being pregnant with Breuer's child. This fantasy was not only an expression of oedipal transference but also an effort to internalize Breuer. Guntrip (1969) described how therapeutic regression may give rise to psychic rebirth: "Nature heals in a state of rest (p. 79). However, there may be both a "regressed ego awaiting

rebirth and unevoked potentialities that have never yet emerged"
(p. 81). If the regression is to a supportive internal object, there is
opportunity for psychic rebirth. Anna O.'s fantasized pregnancy
can be understood as an effort to internalize the ideal object and
bring about the rebirth of the regressed ego. It is the regressed ego's
attachment to the ideal internal object that gives rise to psychic
rebirth. For Anna O., it is the coupling of the oedipal phantasy with
Breuer as the ideal object that gave rise to rebirth.

Unfortunately, Breuer fled from the erotic ramifications of
Anna O.'s fantasy to protect his reputation. His relating to Anna O.
in the I-it mode throughout the treatment may indicate that he not
only feared the erotic transference–counterfransference but defended against the more fundamental I-you mode of therapeutic
symbiosis. Searles (1965) described how intensive therapy with
severely disturbed patients can result in a mutual symbiotic relatedness in which the therapist feels threatened with loss of self and
therefore resists. Most physicians in Breuer's time would not have
dared to become as involved, nor treated a hysteric patient as
humanly, as he. However, his flight from Anna left her emotionally
abandoned and without an object to regress to. The internalization
of the good object was again threatened by rage over the loss of the
external object.

11

THE TREATMENT OF OEDIPAL CONFLICT WITH UNDERLYING ABANDONMENT ANXIETY

This chapter illustrates how the therapist provides interpretations to address neurotic conflicts and offers a holding environment to support underlying ego weakness. Fairbairn believed that Freud, Abraham, and Klein were led astray by the study of melancholia. He believed that Freud had moved away prematurely from the study of hysteria. As the previous chapters demonstrate, the study of melancholia was profitable in leading to the discovery of the depressive position. Yet Fairbairn adopted the slogan "Back to Hysteria" because he felt that the structural situation of hysteria pointed the way to the underlying basis of all psychopathology, the schizoid position. Fairbairn maintained that hysteria was a neurotic defense against schizoid pathology and provided the best avenue to the study of the schizoid core.

THE CLASSICAL THEORY OF HYSTERIA

Classical psychoanalytic theory states that the hysteric patient rejects the object's genitals as a result of the oedipal conflict. This rejection presupposes libidinal attraction. There is a regressive li-

bidinal retreat to orality that becomes manifest by the oral dependent relationship on the external object. This dependence is
maintained as long as the libidinal relationship to the object's
genitals remains repressed. Fairbairn (1954) accepted this description of the dynamics of hysteria but provided a radical change of
emphasis. He stated that the patient repressed the conflicted relationship to the genitals not only to keep the incest taboo but also to
maintain a relationship with the external object through idealization. This idea was based on his theory that the person is primarily
object related and splits off and represses bad or unsatisfactory
aspects of the relationship to the object.

OBJECT RELATIONS THEORY OF HYSTERIA

Object relations theory posits that the hysteric is originally deprived in the relationship to the primary caregiver. There is a
rejection of the breast and the child turns to the father for substitute
mothering. The father is therefore a mother without the exciting
but frustrating breast. However, the phallus becomes a substitute
for the breast. The hysteric's rejecting attitude toward the breast
then persists toward the phallus. The patient relates to the father as
an ideal object as long as the conflict around the phallus remains
split off and repressed (Fairbairn 1941).

Freud (1905) described the dynamics of hysteria as based on
the centrality of the oedipal conflict. Object relations theory perceives the oedipal conflict as the outcome of the earlier conflict of
independence. Splitting and repression are already in effect when
the child is called upon to face the particular conflicts of the oedipal
situation.

THE OEDIPAL CONFLICT AND SPLITTING

The chief novelty that the child encounters in the oedipal phase is
that he is faced with two parental figures as opposed to the one
preoedipal figure. Fairbairn (1944) suggested that the relationship

to the new object, the father, is associated with the same troubling conflicts as described in relation to the original caregiver—that of need, frustration, and rejection. The child utilizes splitting in relation to the father exactly as it had in relationship with the mother. The father is also split into a good and bad object, with the bad object being further divided into an exciting and rejecting object. For Fairbairn, the father is a mother without a breast and the need for the mother underlies the need for the father.

Fairbairn recognized an instinctually based need for the parents during the oedipal phase. The child increasingly recognizes the genital distinction between the parents. Physical needs are directed through the genital channels, the need for the mother including the vagina, the need for the father including the penis. However, Fairbairn emphasized that there is an inverse relationship between the strength of incestuous physical needs and the satisfaction of emotional needs. He said, "The more satisfactory [are the child's] emotional relations with his parents, the less urgent are his physical needs for the genitals" (p. 122).

The child has difficulty managing a relationship with one ambivalently loved object. Faced with two ambivalent relationships, the child finds the situation intolerable and simplifies the situation of two exciting and two rejecting objects by transforming the desired parent into the exciting object and the competing parent into the rejecting object. However, in the background ambivalence persists toward both parents. The child has transformed the relationship to the internal split-off objects into the oedipal situation.

Kernberg (1980) stated that Fairbairn was among the first analysts to understand the connection between preoedipal and oedipal development. However, like Melanie Klein, he had confused the issue by telescoping the oedipal conflict to the earliest months of life. James Grotstein (1981) makes an important contribution in clarifying this confusion. He says that when Klein extended the oedipal conflict to the first year of life, she had in mind a mythic paradigm of thirdness. She was drawing on the oedipal myth to describe a feeding couple in harmony that is disturbed by a third object. This third object is therefore an intruder, a stranger who disrupts the union between baby and mother. This saboteur initially may be the infant's own feelings, its greed, envy, or hostility. It may also be the mother's interest in other objects—reading, talking on the telephone, her attention to herself. Grotstein says that the infant soon personifies the third to be an intruding stranger who is likely to be the father, sibling, or someone else in the mother's life.

Grotstein's idea of the third is similar to Wright's (1991c) concept of the paternal function. Whereas Grotstein stresses the infant's sense of being intruded upon, Wright emphasizes how the infant's identification with the third promotes separation from the mother. Grotstein focuses on the infant's own interpretations of its feelings in creating the third, whereas Wright emphasizes the presence of the actual third. Grotstein and Wright do not have to be viewed as presenting contradictory views, however, but rather as expressing two sides of the paternal function. For this chapter, the importance of the third is that it is an intersection for preoedipal and oedipal development.

In the classical view of the oedipal conflict, the child projects his own aggression onto the rival parent. Seeing the parent through his own projected aggression, the child fears that the parent will retaliate by castrating or rejecting him. Freud (1905) emphasized that it is the child's fear of the parent that motivates him to renounce the oedipal conflict. Edith Jacobson (1964) stated that it is not only out of fear but also out of love for the rival parent that the child renounces incestuous and oedipal wishes. Object relations theory emphasizes that an unresolved oedipal conflict is related to the actual response of the parent. During the oedipal period, the child must experience a sublimated libidinal relationship to the desired parent and a neutralized competitive relationship with the rival parent. The oedipal situation provides an opportunity for growth in the areas of object relations and competition. The two parental objects must neither reject nor overstimulate the child's oedipal love and competitive strivings. Fairbairn (1944) does not make enough of a distinction of the father's role in normative and pathological development. In pathology, the father becomes a substitute for the depriving breast but, as Wright (1991c) points out, in normative development the father has a function in his own right by promoting differentiation from the preoedipal mother. If there is no actual father in the familial situation, it is important for another figure to fill the role of promoting differentiation from fusion.

Guntrip was analyzed by Fairbairn. He (1975) reported that he was surprised that Fairbairn made so many oedipally based interpretations, since he believed that he and Fairbairn were in accord in their views on development. When he brought this issue to Fairbairn's attention, the latter replied that although he believed that the oedipal conflict was the end result and not the primary cause of repression, he nevertheless believed that oedipal issues were of crucial clinical importance. There is often a tendency today to sharply distinguish preoedipal disorders from oedipal neurotic conditions. Because purely neurotic conditions are rarely encountered, the oedipal conflict often receives little attention. In my view, patients that suffer severe preoedipal problems undergo an oedipal conflict, but with a weakened ego. This makes for a more intense oedipal conflict. Similarly, patients with seemingly neurotic disorders often suffer from underlying ego weakness. The following case discussions will illustrate how the therapist provides interpretations of oedipal conflict and a holding relationship for the underlying ego weakness.

THE CASE OF JUSTINE: A DIALECTIC BETWEEN THE OEDIPAL WISH AND TRAUMATIC EXPERIENCE

Background and History

Justine is a patient I (Seinfeld 1990c) discussed in a previous publication from the point of view of separation from symbiosis. I will briefly review her background and proceed to discuss the issues at hand.

Justine is a middle-aged woman who grew up in an intact family, the youngest of three sisters. All of the siblings, including Justine, had histories of psychiatric illness and hospitalization.

Justine's mother was the dominant parental figure. Embittered by her difficult economic situation, she often violently vented her rage on her children. At the same time, she had no activities or work outside the home and was overinvolved with the children, not allowing them to separate. Justine's father was a withdrawn and depressed manual worker. Justine went to him for love and support and to escape the familial chaos and violence. In turn, her love uplifted him from depression. She felt that there had been an escalation of her mother's abusive behavior because of her closeness to her father. When she was 9 years old, her father had fondled her genitals twice.

Justine came to me after having been hospitalized three times for psychiatric care and having had ten years of psychotherapy with different therapists. Her previous therapy was crucial in helping her to stay out of the hospital. She finished college, married, and had a child. The previous therapy was also crucial in enabling her to take care of her child without abusing him. However, her general level of functioning remained minimal.

A Narcissistic Transference

For the first four years of her treatment with me, Justine had an intense, eroticized, ambivalent, dependent transference. She was subject to extreme separation anxiety in the transference and with other significant objects. She abruptly developed a full-blown negative transference through which she separated from the symbiosis. I (Seinfeld 1990c) described this process, which lasted for another four years, in a previous publication. Afterwards, from the eighth through the twelfth year of treatment, she developed a narcissistic transference. She gradually pursued career development and eventually became a full-time professional teacher in a day treatment program for emotionally disturbed children. Her job was demanding and difficult, and she took great pride in her achievements. Larry Josephs (1992) described the importance of empathically accepting the patient's compensatory structures and not always interpreting deep and primitive object relations units. Justine sought mirroring from the self–object transference. I acknowledged her strength and persistence in dealing with a difficult environmental situation. She often said, "No one will help Justine if she doesn't help herself." She was no longer going to be dependent but would put herself first because she was the only one she could count on. I mirrored her autonomy and she gradually developed an idealizing transference. It was my sense that her libidinal need for the exciting object remained split off and repressed and that her excessive antidependent attitude allowed the central self to function autonomously. However, I chose not to interpret this but instead supported the compensatory structures of the central self.

A Deteriorating Environmental Situation

Justine's life situation was complicated by the fact that her young husband suffered from a terminal illness that was diagnosed during the course of her treatment. The husband had taken care of her emotionally and materially, but now there was a change in their roles. Therefore, she was under added pressure to become autonomous and to take care of herself and her family. His situation gradually worsened to the point where he had to stop working. Each year there was an increased threat of him dying suddenly. In the twelfth year of his treatment she was told by physicians that there was a 40 percent chance of sudden death and that his condition was worsening. This situation played a part in the repression of her transference dependence in the interest of functioning.

The Effect of the Reality Situation on the Patient's Internal States

I found that explaining the impact of the reality situation on Justine's internal states helped her to function. The treatment had revealed that she feared to be autonomous because she associated autonomy with abandonment by parental figures. They had kept her dependent and felt injured if she separated. I explained that as she now became increasingly autonomous, her abandonment anxieties were reinforced by the reality situation of her husband becoming more ill as she became more independent. It was as if her autonomy injured him to the point where he would abandon her by dying. It was also necessary to help her to express her ambivalence about the situation. At times when she felt so panicked that she could barely function, I explained that his illness frightened her and made her angry at him for becoming ill, which in turn frightened her and caused her to feel guilty. She acknowledged sometimes wishing he would die so that she could get on with her life, but then she felt sad that he could die without seeing their child grow up and that she would miss him and have to start all over. When she was most panicked, there were underlying murderous feelings toward him that she had to verbalize to calm herself. She felt like a female counterpart to the biblical Job. I provided a holding environment with the provision of concrete services. For instance, I helped her to obtain scholarships so that her child could go away to summer camp, homemaker service while her husband recovered from surgery, and whatever entitlements she was eligible for. On occasion she became self-defeating or unduly frightened of female authorities at work, and I interpreted that she feared the engulfing mother's punishment for separation.

A Crisis Situation

Every year she or her husband took a vacation out of state for a couple of weeks, visiting with one of their parents. Their financial situation did not allow them to go together, but even if her husband went, Justine usually enjoyed the time alone. It was a relief that he was in his parents' care and she was not responsible and did not have to worry. Every morning for the past several years she checked to see if he was still breathing while he slept. The crisis began when her husband took his vacation in the twelfth year of treatment. This time she did not enjoy herself, but instead constantly thought that this is what her life would be like if he died. Thus, instead of feeling that he was on vacation and she was free for a while, she felt as if he had died. She was panicked and her anxiety did not lessen upon his return. It was March and the anxiety spread to the work situation.

The director of the school program was an older, critical, narcissistic woman. Justine had been at the job for a few years and had seen the director fire staff. Justine had been afraid that the director would eventually turn on her and pressure her until she quit. Justine was successful at getting along with the director and had some degree of job security. She was aware that her anxieties were not based on the reality situation but on the director's representation of the abandoning maternal figure. The director was like her mother in that she did not want her staff to be independent and expected them to serve her before themselves or their students.

With the onset of her crisis state, Justine became more fearful of the director. If she committed the slightest infraction or made a mistake, she was certain the director would learn of it and punish her. The director had always been critical, but now Justine became hypersensitive. She was obsessed about every problem that arose in school. She telephoned me for minor problems, feeling that a catastrophe would occur. During the first four years of treatment, she had often called because she had felt disconnected in the transference. However, for the past eight years she rarely called except when faced with a realistic problem. Her anxiety now spread in the work situation. There were a number of students who were known to have been sexually abused. Whenever she saw them, she panicked for no apparent reason. A male aide was accused of sexually molesting a student, and she became obsessed with the fear that she would be falsely accused of sexual abuse. Her anxiety and depression became so severe that she could barely go to work. I had spoken to her when the panic began about seeing a psychopharmacologist and she now agreed to go. The psychopharmacologist empathized with the severity of her emotional condition and the precariousness of her life situation and agreed to see her at a very reduced fee and to be available for phone contacts to monitor the medication. He placed her on antidepression medication.

Management

Justine felt so upset that she stopped going to work. I encouraged her to return as soon as possible. She felt pressured. She said that she doubted if she could ever return and that this meant that her family could not eat, that she had failed them, and that she might as well kill herself. She was in conflict about going to a hospital but decided she did not want to. The psychopharmacologist and I remained in contact monitoring her day-to-day condition. She could barely get out of bed. There were brief periods when she felt better and thought of returning to work. She panicked, fearing she might collapse in her classroom. Given her past psychiatric history and her vulnerability, I thought she could collapse on the job. Therefore I no longer recommended that she return directly to work but rather encouraged her to wait until she felt more assured and less worried and to allow for some time to rest and recuperate. The psychopharmacologist advised her to allow for some time for the medication to work and said that he would give her a note when she was ready to return. She worried that she might not return for a long time and wondered how would she manage. In my countertransference I felt as if she were planning not to return. However, I refrained from reacting and joined her in discussing what motions she could take to support herself or prevent financial disaster. We discussed how she might declare bankruptcy, go on disability, take a leave of absence, enter a new line of work. She stated that her husband was panicked that she'd never return to work and sometimes treated her like a malingerer. At such times, she felt suicidal. She was angry at him for pressuring her, saying that she had stood by him throughout his long illness but that he could only blame her. She also worried that her upset state would make him more ill. He did not want therapeutic help for himself but met with me on occasion and felt better after venting his concerns. He was then more supportive of her.

During this period Justine called nearly every day and came in for twice weekly sessions. She felt that she had worked so hard all these years in therapy in vain. I acknowledged how hard she had worked but said that the feeling that things would never be better, that she'd never get back to work, was not a reliable guide because it reflected how she felt now. After a number of weeks, once she had rested and the medication had taken effect, she would feel differently and would see things differently. The psychopharmacologist also advised her that the medication would eventually serve to insulate her from the intensity of the depression and anxiety but that she would still have bad days and would need to work out her problems in therapy.

When Justine felt suicidal, it was helpful for her to put these impulses into words, assuring me that she would not act on them. She described how she felt like cutting her wrist, throwing herself out a window, swallowing all of her medication. She feared that I would panic, not trust her, and call the police. If she conveyed any doubt about controlling her suicidal impulses, I stated that for us to work together on an outpatient basis, there had to be mutual trust. If she could not guarantee her cooperation, she needed to be in a hospital for her own protection. She promised she would call me or the psychopharmacologist and go to a hospital and not hurt herself. She reminded me that in the twelve years she had been seeing me, she had never made a suicidal gesture or attempt. By helping her vent her suicidal impulses, I was following Freud's recommendation that the patient should put feelings into words and not actions. By calming the anxiety she evoked in me, I helped her to contain the destructive feelings.

Winnicott (1955) described symptomatic children and adults needing a period of rest and regression at home to provide protection from impingement. The therapist's function during this process is to provide management. Justine wondered what brought on the crisis and concluded that stress had an accumulative effect on her. I had always acknowledged the severe stress of her environmental situation. She felt that her environmental situation would not improve in the foreseeable future. It would not change until her husband died. Sometimes she wished it would happen already, but then it may be worse and she'd have new problems. She could see no light at the end of the tunnel. During this period of regression I rarely made interpretations. However, I did point out that she had been living with the stress of her husband's dying and a difficult environmental situation for several years. She had found these manageable though difficult, so it was possible that there was something else going on. She wondered what and I said that I was not yet sure but it would be worthwhile for us to think about it. I acknowledged that there was cumulative effect but said that the problems had been accumulating for several years. Perhaps it was the effect of the stress on her internal state, or what her internal state made of the stress, that we needed to think about.

A Bridge between the External Situation and the Internal State

After three weeks, Justine felt well enough to return to work. However, her symptoms remained severe. She felt bleak about her future and had extreme anxiety attacks for no apparent reason. She had no intention of doing anything now, but she said she had always had the feeling that she would eventually kill herself. On occasion, she found herself distressed about the same things that troubled her shortly before she had stopped working. At this point, I began to interpret her anxieties while continuing to provide holding as needed.

I acknowledged the realistic stressors in her life but added that her ability to cope with them was undermined by internal emotional issues that we needed to understand. At times she could see this but more often she believed that her emotional state was based solely on her reality situation. However, believing all of her troubles were due to her external situation made her feel worse because there was no way to quickly change that. If I encouraged her to explore her inner state, she shot back, "There is nothing further to explore. You don't know what it's like to have a sick husband at home. That is my problem." I invited her to tell me, adding that external and internal factors did not have to contradict one another. She cried and ventilated about her life situation, then calmed down, saying that she did not mean to snap at me. I said, "External stress itself could be unmanageable, and your life comes close to qualifying as that, but if there is any way to explore your inner situation—what you are making of your life situation, not only what it is making of you—it may be worth doing." She could see that she had lived with her situation for a long time and that there may be more to it than she understood, but she did not know where to begin.

An opportunity for exploration arose shortly thereafter. She mentioned feeling panicked about a girl in her class whom she knew to be sexually abused by her mother's boyfriend. She became obsessed with this and similar situations. She also expressed relief that the female director left her alone since she returned to work, but she was worried that she would start with her and try to fire her.

Freud (1905) described how certain trains of thought that become exaggerated have an obsessive quality and are not under the volitional control of the patient. Justine knew her worries were irrational, yet she could not be rid of them. I commented that she had become anxious seeing a number of girls who had been abused and about the male school aide who had been accused of abusing a child. She replied that whenever she saw them she thought of herself and her father. I remarked that they represent her relationship with her father and the severity of her anxiety shows that that relationship is still active and alive in her mind. Justine then referred to her father's sexualized relationship with her. She said, "We spoke about this in the past, but I guess it's still an issue."

I interpreted that the female director represented her mother, whom she had described as abusing her for her relationship with her father. I pointed out that even when the female director is not criticizing her, Justine nevertheless expects or imagines her to be criticizing her. I said, "You are having the internal mother, represented by the female director, attack you." I added that the director was a perfect person to represent the internal mother because she was critical and narcissistic like the mother. In this way, I demonstrated that the relationships to her father and to her mother existed in her mind. I added that her internal mother was attacking her for the relationship she had with her father. I interpreted the oedipal conflict but not exclusively in terms of memories, wishes, and defenses.

Justine went into detail about how her mother had abused her. The mother had always been abusive but became more so as Justine became closer to her father. The mother had never openly protested but was always angry. Justine wondered why this inner situation was awakened at this time.

The Oedipal Conflict and Anxiety over Success

Justine said that for the first time in her life, she had been successful, working in a respected and challenging position and supporting herself and her family. The job required that she take courses toward a master's degree. She had tried over the last couple of years but had felt overwhelmed by the work added onto her other responsibilities and had dropped the courses. Other than that, she had been successful at everything she tried over the past several years and felt better able to cope with life. She therefore did not understand why she became depressed and anxious again to the point of collapsing. I replied that it might be the very success that she was beginning to experience that resulted in her emotional collapse. I explained that the first struggle for success in her childhood would have been in competing with her mother and sisters for the affection of her father. I pointed out that in her family, the natural struggle for success has been complicated by her father's actually fondling her. She then perceived her mother's abuse as a punishment for the "success." I remarked that it is likely that, for her, success is now associated with something forbidden—the incestuous tie to the father and the retaliation of the mother. The fact that she was now having some success in her life could be awakening this conflict.

This interpretation did not have any immediate effect on ameliorating the conflict. I made it to provide an explanatory, educational frame of reference for future transference interpretations. Winnicott (1972) also described how playing around with ideas may provide relief for the fragile patient from overwhelmingly intense affective experience. Justine responded to this explanation by playing around with the idea of fear of success and the many ways people may be wrecked by success. It seemed that there was a temporary respite from her overwhelming anxiety and depression.

The Response to Loss

The situation of her husband's illness reinforced early anxieties. Justine felt that she could not do what was required of her to take care of herself. I now brought up the idea that the onset of her current symptom occurred when her husband took a short vacation. She had imagined what it would be like if he were dead and had panicked. We had established that she grew up fearing autonomy because it was associated with being abandoned by her mother. When she tried to be independent, her mother acted injured and angry and withdrew. I said, "If you prepare to take care of yourself and your child, you are preparing for your husband's death, and it feels as if you are bringing about the loss. If you do not prepare, then maybe he will know you still need him and will not abandon you. He represents the mother who abandons you if you are autonomous."

She often complained of feeling engulfed by having to take care of her husband, abused when he took out his anger on her, and frightened. I reminded her of how she had felt engulfed, abused, and frightened by her mother while acknowledging the realistic hardships of living with her ill husband. I also pointed out that when she imagined him to be dead and that she was on her own, it felt as if she had lost him and was in mourning—that she was preparing for his death by anticipatory mourning.

The Escape from the Persecutory Preoedipal Mother to the Idealized Father

Justine observed and projected anger into her husband. There was the vicious cycle of her fear of losing him giving rise to anger at him for leaving her and his anger at his illness reinforcing her projection of anger into him. When she was young and became disturbed by her mother, she was able to go to her father for comfort. I said that her need for the father was reawakened by the impending loss of her husband, which in itself was a reliving of the fear of abandonment and abuse by the mother. I said it was this need for the father that prompted the disturbing thoughts about the sexually abused children and abusing authorities at school.

She responded by describing how she had crawled into her father's bed as a child and how he had held and comforted her. She felt soothed and protected from the violence and chaos of her family. Then the fondling occurred. She felt it was her fault that he fondled her because she had returned to his bed. She knew it was wrong, but it felt pleasurable. Lying close to him not only felt comforting but sensual. She had always felt that she had seduced him into touching her. She was not angry at him, nor did she blame him. After the second occurrence, he never fondled her again. She therefore felt that on some level he cared or at least knew what he did was wrong.

Antilibidinal Retaliation

During her workday she was busy enough not to be distracted by the thoughts of her father. After work, though, she was obsessed, remembering the incidents as if reliving them. It was by the very vividness and intensity of such experiences that I was able to demonstrate that the relationship to her father was still alive and active in her psyche. I said, "Your actual father died over a decade ago. Yet the intensity of your anxiety is in proportion to how you would feel if this were occurring now. It is not only a memory you suffer from but also the relationship to your father and all the wishes, fears, and feelings associated with it that remain alive and active now." As she relived the incidents with her father, it was necessary for her to call me for support. The memories of her father brought on self-destructive thoughts. She needed to describe those thoughts to obtain relief. I allowed her to put them into words as long as she assured me she wouldn't act on them. If she would act on them, she needed to be hospitalized. I interpreted that the self-destructive impulses reflected her identification with the mother abusing her for her actions with the father.

Freud (1914) described how the patient abandons herself to a compulsion to repeat, which replaces the recollection of significant but repressed memories. In the compulsion to repeat, the patient reproduces symptoms that are transformed into pieces of real life: actions, character traits, inhibitions, fantasies, feelings, which are not always harmless if acted out. Freud remarked that as the patient lives through the past as something real and accurate, the therapist must tolerate the inevitable repetition but also gradually translate it back to the terms of the past. Freud stated that the transference was the means the therapist has for curbing the patient's compulsion to repeat or act out. The handling of the transference may allow for the compulsion to repeat to assert itself harmlessly within limits. Freud said, "We admit it into the transference as to a playground, in which it is allowed to let itself go in almost complete freedom and is required to display before us all the pathogenic impulses hidden in the depths of the patient's mind" (p. 374). Freud described the transference as an intermediary realm between illness and real life through which the therapist helps the patient transform repetition into recollection.

The Emergence of the Transference

An external incident brought to the fore the intensity of the transference. A driver of a car lost control in Washington Square Park, injuring and killing some people. Justine knew that my office was near the park and that I was often in the area. She left messages on all of my phone machines, fearing that I had been injured or killed. She became aware of how dependent she felt, saying that if it had not been for me, she would have thrown herself out a window long ago. She said that she was only able to withstand the stress of her husband's illness and her own emotional disturbance with my support. She thought that her feelings about me were involved in what she was going through about her father. I had tried interpreting this earlier, but to no avail. I now remarked that her ambivalent relationship to her mother gave rise to the need for her father in childhood. She now relived the ambivalence toward her mother in the relationship to her husband, and she turned toward the father in the transference. I explained that I was not referring to myself personally, but rather to what I stood for in the transference. As this theme developed, she acknowledged it sometimes. At other times she stated that she felt an erotic dependence on other men, such as the psychopharmacologist, her child's doctor, or a male director on the job. I pointed out that they were all authority figures or helpers and there was the possibility that she displaced transference feelings onto them because she was much less involved and therefore safer. I reminded her of how intense the transference was for the first four years of treatment and how excited, frustrated, and angry she had felt. I reiterated that the feelings were not about me personally but about what I represent, her father. I said she may displace the transference feelings so that she could relate to me in an idealized way without being overly disturbed by excitement, frustration, or anger. I reminded her of how much she said she needed me and that it was the very intensity of this need that accounted for her efforts to maintain me as all good or ideal.

Once she had integrated these thoughts, I remarked that she had repressed the exciting and frustrating aspects of the transference over a long while, which helped her to function and to use the therapy. This was fine. If it continued in the same way, there would be no reason to raise this issue of transference. The problem was that where she was in her treatment—the feelings of ambivalence and loss about her husband/mother, the conflicts over success—the transference feelings were brought to the fore as symptoms of anxiety and depression.

The Emergence of Rage at the Abusive Father
in the Transference

Justine acknowledged that when she thought of her father, she thought of me. I said, "Your father died long ago. The reason thinking of that relationship panics you is that the feelings remain alive in the transference. When you become very anxious, the danger is not that you want to act on these feelings with your actual dead father but rather that you fear acting on them with the living father in the transference."

As she became aware of the transference, she realized that her panic attacks were the result of anger at her father. She felt that he did not care enough about her to protect her. He acted on his own needs at her expense. She realized this through her wish that I act out with her sexually and understood that if I were to, it would mean I did not care about her or her treatment. She could not continue to be angry, but instead blamed herself for going to her father's bed. I remarked that her dilemma was that she had needed him, that he was the only nurturing parent she had.

Fairbairn (1943) described how the abused child often remains loyal to the abusing parent by internalizing and identifying with the parent's negative attributes. I pointed out that a child needs the parent whether that parent is good or bad. Her father was also the only giving parent. She therefore imagined him to be all good and giving by blaming herself. I noted that she had continued the same pattern with me by idealizing our relationship and repressing feelings of excitement that would give rise to frustration and anger.

Eliciting Transference Fantasy

The interpretations calmed her to a degree, but she still felt to blame. She believed it was because the wishes still were active in the transference. I asked her to directly describe them, explaining that doing so may help to clarify the reason for her anxiety, self-blame, and conflicts over success and autonomy. She feared being overwhelmed with anxiety if she fully discussed her transferential feelings. However, she also feared feeling worse if she did not deal with them. I replied that she only recently returned to work and it would not be good for her symptoms to worsen. I suggested that we look at why she was afraid instead of going directly into what she feared. She said that she feared trying to seduce me. She had been in treatment with me for twelve years and felt she knew me well enough to know I valued her treatment and would protect it. However, because of what occurred with her father, there was a nagging fear that she would succeed. I remarked on her use of the word "succeed" and related it to our earlier discussions of how success at school or work was forbidden because it symbolized incestuous success with the father. She then said it is likely she would not succeed with me and then would feel depressed and rejected. She felt that either way, she would lose.

I said that her need for her father was complicated by her unsatisfactory relationship to her mother. Not receiving the maternal care she needed, she turned to the father for substitute mothering. I explained that a child naturally experiences sensual feelings toward both parents at being held. There is also a wish to compete for and win the parent. It is sensual and emotional. Justine recalled thinking of her father as the most handsome man on earth. She had romantic feelings for him and fantasized marrying him when she grew up. I interpreted that the natural sensual feelings toward her father were made urgent by the earlier deprivation at the hands of her mother and the sexual abuse and overstimulation by her father. This interpretation was made on the basis of Ferenczi's (1933) theory that the child's natural infantile sexuality registered in the language of tenderness is transformed into the language of passion by the parent's overstimulating behavior. Also influential was Fairbairn's (1941) theory that, in the oedipal phase, the child experiences a libidinal need with a genital component for the parent as a whole object, but that the need for the parent may be channeled exclusively into the genital area and the parent related to as a part-object when the general emotional relationship is unsatisfactory.

Justine said that she felt like coming over to me and being held, as her father had held her, especially when she was frightened or distressed. She imagined we would undress one another. She had a wish to touch my penis and recalled having the same wish as a child lying next to her father. She imagined performing fellatio. Intercourse would follow, but it was the fellatio that she longed for. She was extremely anxious while describing these fantasies but felt relieved afterwards. The relief was identical to how she felt after putting her suicidal or aggressive feelings into words. We met twice weekly, on a Saturday and on a weekday. She wanted to restrict the discussion of her transferential wishes to the Saturday session because she feared that discussing them on a weekday would provoke too much anxiety and might interfere with her functioning at work. However, she found that after not discussing the transference on the weekday she became more anxious and had to call me for support. She found that when she discussed her transferential feelings on the following weekday, she was relieved and did not need to call. She was also able to transfer her libidinal feelings to her husband and enjoy greater intimacy with him.

The Discovery of the Maternal Transference Underlying the Paternal Transference

Justine said that during the first years of treatment when she had experienced an intense erotic transference, she would have acted on it even if it destroyed her treatment. She depended completely on me to set limits and protect her treatment. Now she felt that the treatment was more important than the pleasure she would have from acting out. She herself wanted to protect the treatment. This made her feel sad, pained, and frustrated. I likened it to mourning— giving up the oedipal wishes toward her father—and to anticipatory grief regarding the loss of her husband. She said there was a deeper factor. She felt the same way when she endured a postpartum depression. She discontinued breast feeding because she felt that the baby was depriving her of blood and life, not only milk. She did not feel comfortable as a mother because she had not been mothered. In the transference there is not only excitement and sexuality but also comforting and an escape from the burdens of life. Justine felt that there was something about mothering in her sexual fantasies. She likened the fellatio fantasy to nursing at the breast and concluded that she was feeling the pain of giving up the need for the father and the mother. There was a quality of mourning, but of even greater significance was a feeling of longing that could never be fulfilled.

Rage in the Transference

At around this time, I was planning a monthlong vacation. For Justine, this loss became condensed with the earlier loss of her father and the impending loss of her husband. Intellectually, she believed I had a right to go on vacation, but emotionally she felt that if I really cared, I would not go away for so long, given what she had been going through since March. As she verbalized the erotic fantasies, she became enraged because I frustrated her by sitting and listening or providing interpretations instead of actions.

As Wright (1991d) states, by responding to the patient with empathy and attunement, the therapist becomes the object of the patient's earliest unfulfilled needs. The two-person empathic relationship heightens feelings of intimacy and revives the earliest longings for the mother. In Fairbairn's (1944) terms, the object is transformed from a good to an exciting object. Furthermore, the therapist does not then respond with literal holding but assumes the paternal function in providing an interpretation. The exciting object is transformed into a rejecting object. Wright maintains that if the therapist did no more than recapitulate the earlier maltreatment inflicted on the patient by his original parental objects, it is doubtful that the patient would remain in treatment. Somehow the therapist must convey to the patient not only the distant paternal function of provision of the word but also the caring, empathic, maternal function.

In the treatment of Justine, I explicitly acknowledged the difficult position she assumed by putting all of her feelings and thoughts concerning the transference into words, while I just sat and listened or provided interpretations in order to protect her treatment. I also remarked on her efforts to help herself and her valuing of her treatment in assuming such a difficult position. Expressing her libidinal dependent wishes, she became aware of her frustration and rage, both because I sat and listened and because I was leaving for vacation. She verbalized impulses to cut off my

penis, come in with a knife to stab me, shoot me, and organize all of
my patients to protest against my departure. Verbalizing her rage
provided the same relief as verbalizing sexual, dependent, or suicidal feelings. In becoming enraged at me, she also became more
aware of her rage at her father. She was aware of rage because he
abused her, but also because he stimulated and excited her without
culminating the act and therefore rejecting her. Fairbairn (1954)
remarked that the child is made to feel more rejected by the parental
object's overstimulation.

Justine relived the rage at her father as she became enraged in
the transference as her libidinal, dependent needs were excited by
the therapist's empathy but frustrated by interpretations. She found
that if she became angry at the therapist, she could be angry at her
father. When she could not be angry at the therapist, she could not
be angry at her father. It was exceedingly difficult to hold onto
positive feelings about the therapist or her father when she was
angry at them. However, she continually worked at doing so.
Justine was aware that although her father abused her, he was also
the figure in her early life from whom she felt love. Thus feeling
good about herself was intrinsically tied to feeling good about him.
If she decided that he was all bad, that the love he showed her was of
no value, merely a sham, it would mean that the only experience in
her early life of being loved, upon which rested her core self-worth,
was of no value. She would be unlovable and worthless.

Jacobson (1965) described how, in early development, self and
object representations are split off into exclusively libidinal and
exclusively aggressive self and object sets. What this means is that
when Justine viewed her father as utterly rejecting, she invariably
felt worthless and utterly rejected, whereas when she viewed him as
utterly loving and accepting, she invariably felt loved and utterly
accepted. Treatment now focused on helping her to integrate her
relationships with the father who was giving, caring, and nurturing
with the father who abused, excited, and frustrated her, who did
not care enough about her not to abuse her. The idealizing transference protected her from facing this dilemma. At the same time, a
prolonged idealizing transference was necessary to strengthen the
internal ideal object so that it would not be overwhelmed by the
repressed and split-off exciting and rejecting objects.

In writing of transference love, Freud (1915) said,

> With one type of woman, to be sure, this attempt to preserve the love transference for the purposes of analytic work without gratifying it will not succeed. These are women of an elemental passionateness; they tolerate no surrogate; they are children of nature who refuse to accept the spiritual instead of the material; to use then poet's words, they are amenable only to the "logic of gruel and the argument of dumplings." With such people one has the choice either to return their love or else to bring down upon oneself the full force of the mortified woman's fury. In neither event can one safeguard the interests of the treatment. One must acknowledge failure and withdraw; and at leisure study the problem how the capacity for neurosis can be combined with such an intractable craving for love [p. 386].

It seems that the urgent libidinal craving described by Freud is the result of an unsatisfactory relationship in early life giving rise to an exclusive channeling of libidinal need into a genital relationship to an exciting part-object. A therapeutic approach that combines interpretation addressed to these dynamics and a supportive object relationship may provide a somewhat more favorable prognosis, although the treatment remains difficult.

A RETREAT FROM OEDIPAL COMPETITION

This second clinical vignette illustrates how the therapist analyzes a patient's retreat from the oedipal conflict to anality in object relational terms. Fred was an adult patient working for over ten years on a doctoral dissertation in philosophy. He described his familial situation as follows: his mother was a depressed, highly critical women who pervasively devalued whatever he achieved. His father was a highly narcissistic man who inherited wealth but failed at several businesses. He demanded that the son admire him but showed little interest in his son's interests. The patient always felt that his father never allowed him to compete. The father seemingly had great admiration for highly educated persons. However, if such a person ever failed, the father was quick to pronounce that all the book learning in the world added up to little common sense. Fred was always an excellent student. Although the father took pleasure boasting about his son's high grades, he had little interest in the subject matter he studied.

Fred complained that he could not work on his dissertation. Whenever he tried to work, he thought of the dissertation committee and imagined that they would reject it. When I inquired about the work he was doing, he described it as too complex and technical to go into but that it was of great importance. Over time, he described his work in rather grandiose terms, imagining that other people would be either too ignorant to understand or too envious to appreciate his work. He did not tell anyone about it because he imagined they would spoil it by their negative reaction. I recognized the same theme in other areas of his life. He said that when he went out with a woman he felt anxious and blocked. His mind was abuzz with brilliant thoughts, but he feared that if he expressed them, the other person may not be interested. I connected the similarity in theme in his work efforts and his relationship with women. I said, "You are trying to keep the contents of your mind as good as gold and you fear that if you express them, they will be transformed into shit."

He was interested in my comments, so I said that putting his contents out, expressing himself, may seem risky in that he had not had much experience with people appreciating his achievements or products. Fred said that when he had produced anything for his parents, it had been treated like shit and rejected. That is how it felt with his dissertation. I said that so long as the ideas remained in his mind, he could feel that they were as good as gold. If he put them out into the world and someone criticized them, he would feel that they had been turned into shit. Fred said that the problem was that it is inevitable that his work will be criticized—it is part of the committee process. He said, "I have read other dissertations and most are full of shit. They are terribly boring and not of great value—at least some that I've read. The persons I know who finished accepted the criticisms, made the recommended changes—they did not give up."

> *Therapist*: (laughing) So what you are suggesting is that working on a dissertation requires throwing around shit—a kind of

playing in shit—and that your need to keep your ideas as good as gold prevents this play.

Fred: This makes me laugh. Do you know I always call my parents pieces of shit? I call everyone that. Either that or asshole. My parents made me feel like a piece of shit.

Therapist: You imagine that if you put out your ideas to the committee, they will reject them. Thinking this makes you feel shitty about yourself and them.

Patient: This is not only true about the committee, it's true with everyone.

Therapist: The fear is that if you express your ideas, feelings—your inner products—you and they will be found shitty. This is what happened between you and your parents. What you put out was spoiled, turned into shit, and you found them to be shitty parents, or pieces of shit as you say. Therefore, you keep your thoughts to yourself and they remain as good as gold. Then you don't have to relive the shitty feelings regarding your parents. By keeping your thoughts, you also hold onto your parents.

Fred feared completing his dissertation. In this society, a Ph.D. signifies success, power, achievement, prestige. Thus, for Fred, the Ph.D. signified the phallus. If he earned it, his father would be jealous. His natural, competitive oedipal strivings were complicated by the fact that his father felt depressed and defeated by life. Freud (1915b) said that the oedipally competing child projects his aggression onto the father, then fears that the father will retaliate by castrating him. The oedipal situation becomes overloaded if the rival parent is in reality burdened by the child's competition. Borrowing Ferenczi's (1933) language about sexuality, we could say that the parent's aggression and jealousy is grafted onto the child's natural aggression and competitiveness. Fred's mother always complained about the father's failures. For Fred, finishing the Ph.D. unconsciously meant winning his mother's love and defeating his father. He retreated from the oedipal conflict to that of anality. The prized Ph.D. disintegrated into anal fragments that were idealized as gold so that they were not devalued and turned into shit. However, feces were the psychosexual symbol of the patient's relationship to the parents as inner contents. Anal retentiveness thereby served the idealization of Fred's relationship to the mothering object to avoid separation, abandonment and oedipal competition.

THE DIALECTIC BETWEEN OEDIPAL AND
PREOEDIPAL CONFLICT

George Frank (personal communication 1980) described how borderline patients typically vacillate from oedipal competition to
rapprochement conflicts around separation and abandonment. The
patient takes a small step toward competing, is panicked by fear of
punishment, and retreats to a position of fearing being abandoned
by the preoedipal object. Symbiotic clinging ensues to avoid abandonment. It seems that competing with an oedipal rival as a separate
object gives rise to a fear of punishment by the oedipal rival, which
is transformed into a fear of abandonment by the preoedipal object.
The retreat from oedipal conflict is immediately followed by the
symbiotic clinging to the preoedipal rival as a result of abandonment anxiety.

John's father died at the beginning of the oedipal phase. He
developed an overly dependent relationship with his mother. As an
adolescent, he failed most of his subjects and dropped out of school.
As a result of therapy, he entered a special vocational training
program and began to apply himself. At around this time, he
became infatuated with a local girl. She responded with interest and
they began to date. At this same time, John became preoccupied
with a neighborhood bully. The bully picked on John as he picked
on many neighborhood youngsters. John became obsessed with
thinking that the bully had it in for him. He became so preoccupied
with the bully that he began to neglect his vocational training. The
girlfriend was very ambivalent about a relationship. One week she
expressed interest in John, but the next week she avoided him. He
could not recognize that she had her own conflicts about intimacy,
but instead felt that her avoidance was a reflection on him. He
increasingly neglected his schooling as he became increasingly
preoccupied with the persecution by the local bully and the girlfriend's avoidant behavior. Feeling rejected, he called her daily,
pleading with her to see him. He learned she was dating another boy
and became extremely jealous. She spoke to John on the phone but
would not see him. He imagined that he lost her because he was a
failure. In his preoccupation with her, he discontinued going to his
training classes and all other constructive activities in his life.

John's attendance at the vocational school and his relationship with the girlfriend reflected increased autonomy and oedipal competitive strivings as a result of his therapy. The girlfriend's ambivalent behavior was similar to that of his mother. Thus his relationship with her expressed oedipal strivings but also an increased need for the preoedipal mother as he became more separate from the actual mother. The bully he became preoccupied with represented a return of the oedipal father whom he feared would punish him for his newly expressed oedipal wishes. He gradually retreated from oedipal conflict as he stopped going to the vocational training program. He increasingly related to the girlfriend as an abandoning preoedipal mother. He transformed her from an oedipal to a preoedipal object by focusing entirely on her distancing reactions and ignoring her more accepting, loving responses. By perceiving her distancing behavior as rejecting because of his worthlessness, he raised the specter of the abandoning object that he then clung to. The patient unconsciously attributed the death of his father in early childhood to his own rivalrous wishes. It was this situation as well as the exciting and rejecting behavior on the part of his mother that set the stage for his later conflicts.

In the treatment of such patients, Frank recommends focusing interpretations of the oscillation or movement between the oedipal competitiveness and the preoedipal depressive position. The therapist should interpret the patient's retreat from the anxiety of competitiveness or autonomy. Anxiety is associated with change, entering new territory, and facing the unknown. Depression is uncomfortable but is safe because it is known. In depression there is a feeling of not going anywhere, of being stuck. There is a berating of the self for being lazy, for not changing, for being inadequate. The sense of being stuck is that of being stuck with the bad object. The self-disparagement is followed by self-pity and self-indulgence. It is as if the patient tries to be autonomous and competitive and the bad object warns of danger, punishment, abandonment. There is a retreat from the subsequent anxiety. The bad object then accuses the patient of laziness, a lack of motivation, and inadequacy. When the patient is sufficiently discouraged, the bad object shows pity saying, "Don't worry, I still love you. No matter how much of a failure you are, I will not abandon you. In fact, you are such a failure that I am the only one who could ever love you. Therefore, you had better stay with me. It's all right if you don't go to school or work or meet new persons. Who could blame you? Have a drink or some drugs. I understand." Thus self-pity is followed by self-indulgence.

The above clinical vignettes illustrate the importance of the oedipal conflict from an object relations viewpoint. Although it is no longer considered the ultimate basis of psychopathology, it nevertheless remains crucial to development. The existence of early object relations disturbance often affects the later outcome of the oedipal phase and early splitting underlies the oedipal configuration as described by Fairbairn (1944).

12

INTERNALIZING A CONTAINING OBJECT

The patient, Edward, is a businessman in his thirties. He came to therapy because former girlfriends and wives complained that he did not share feelings, had little psychological insight, and could not give emotionally. Edward was married twice. His first wife complained of his detachment and miserliness with money. He went to a therapist to appease her. He could find nothing to discuss, was blocked, and gained little insight. When his first wife left, he quit therapy. The therapist interpreted that Edward attempted to make her feel abandoned as he had been made to feel abandoned by his wife. Edward did not feel abandoned consciously and concluded that the therapist felt abandoned. When girlfriends and a second wife had identical complaints, he began to wonder if they were correct. However, he was confused because he was always generous with his time and money.

PERSONAL HISTORY

Edward grew up in an intact, wealthy family. He had an older sister and a younger brother. The siblings were married and successful professionals. Although he was successful in his career, he felt he had surrendered center stage to his siblings. His brother was a known professional athlete and was very self-assured. His sister was a nationally known, highly respected attorney. A cousin, Jennifer, had lived with the family after the death of her parents. She was Edward's age and he thought of her as a half-sister. Jennifer was the only person Edward ever spoke to about his problems. She now lived alone and was depressed and lonely and sometimes called Edward for comfort. Edward was the most socially outgoing among his siblings. He was never aware of this until he was in treatment. His siblings had no personal friends and only knew people through business activities. Edward was not sociable, by any standard, but he did have some friends and took part in school activities.

Edward described his mother as a removed and self-absorbed woman. She met the material needs of her family but did not provide emotional support. If the children came to her with problems, she said, "Oh, come—you're not really upset. I know that can't really bother you." Edward and his siblings complied. His cousin Jennifer remained troubled by the loss of her parents and problems at school. She returned home crying and complaining that peers picked on her. The mother said, "Can't you leave me alone? You're so sensitive. What is it you want? What is wrong with you? There are enough problems to deal with. Act your age and quit being a baby." The parents could not tolerate Jennifer and sent her to live with other relatives.

Edward's father was described as a highly narcissistic man. He had been extremely successful in business and local politics. He insisted that his children keep company only with youth from wealthy families. The father expressed a familial chauvinism, claiming they were superior in beauty, brains, and blood. The parents also referred to one another as the very best mother and the very best father. The father said, "Isn't your mother the very best? Look at everything she does."

Edward described his adolescence as uneventful. He performed adequately in high school and college. He joined up with local athletic and recreational activities and was friends with local peers. He was neither enthusiastic or troubled by the events in his life.

There was one incident he recalled being excited about. He went on a camping trip with his senior class and met his first girlfriend. He was excited about being on his own, being with his first girl, exploring new territory. He described this adventure in our first session and clearly came to life. This liveliness was in contrast to his ordinary emotional constriction. He felt his life to be dull and uneventful. He had friends that he did things with. They played sports, camped out, and more recently went to a bar for a beer and to watch a game.

In his love relationships with women he felt that he could neither commit himself nor separate. There was one woman he lived with for a couple of years. He provided for her materially and was agreeable about doing whatever she asked, but neither of them felt any emotional bond. He felt that it was time to end the relationship but feared he would hurt her feelings. They could not decide to separate. They both had affairs. He realized that she became involved with someone to make him jealous. He was only a little upset but pretended he was more upset than he was. She was pleased and for a time they felt closer, but then it went back to how it was. She had a second affair to end their relationship. He wondered why he did not leave her. He felt it was an expression of his problem, never to take the initiative.

In his first marriage, he thought that his wife was hysterical and demanding. He worried about money and making ends meet. She complained that he was cheap and cared only for money. He felt she was unsympathetic to his financial concerns. He earned a good living but could not live beyond his means. He did not feel that she was greedy for his money, but rather that she did not know its value. As their marriage ended, he was more concerned with losing money than with losing her. He knew that his worry was not realistic because she was not financially minded and did not fight the settlement.

In his second marriage, Edward became more aware of his difficulties with intimacy. The second wife had identical complaints as the first one concerning his detachment and lack of spontaneous feeling. She did not have a tendency toward hysteria, nor was she excessively demanding. Nevertheless, he did not feel emotionally connected and began to recognize his problems. After they had been married four years, she developed a terminal illness and died within a year. He completely devoted himself to taking care of her but actually felt little sadness over losing her. There were fleeting moments when grief overcame him, but then he became numb. He could not feel for her suffering. He recognized that the momentary feeling of grief had more to do with himself and an infantile terror over being left alone. As she lay dying, he became obsessed with expenses. He felt guilty about his lack of concern and began to consider therapy.

The second wife had been dead for a year and he lived alone. He went through the motions of living, but with little vitality. At work he did his job but avoided socializing. Friends and family left messages on his answering machine, but he did not reply. He felt basically uninterested in people. His colleagues sometimes invited him out for a drink, but he never went. He wondered what was lacking—was he antihuman, without ordinary feelings for people? It was at this point that he came for treatment. He was quite tentative in his request, saying he wished to try only a couple of sessions.

THE BEGINNING PHASE

In the beginning of treatment, Edward repeatedly voiced anxiety over having nothing to say. He discussed the problems and his history and expressed concerns that he was not delving into deep matters, only the everyday past and present facts of his life. I responded that such issues are important in their own right and that the deep issues are not tapped until the groundwork is done. I said, "They are not reached by a strained effort. It is best to go into whatever is on your mind, even if it seems trivial, irrelevant, and superficial, and let the deep things come of their own accord."

When he expressed anxiety that he would not have anything to say, I did not explore or interpret resistance, but instead provided holding: "So far, you have had things to say." He acknowledged having more to say than expected and I said, "It is my sense that there has been something to say, so why shouldn't it continue?"

THE SELF AS OBJECT

Edward's narrative suggested that he experienced his sense of self as more an object than a subject. Feelings, thoughts, and life events were depicted as happening to him rather than being created by him. Ogden (1986) pointed out that the client who experiences himself as an object lacks the capacity to symbolize and relates on a concrete level with little insight. Thus, if Edward described how a woman was angry at him because he did not share his feelings or have insight, I did not interpret his fear of intimacy or withholding as aggression, but instead remarked upon his dilemma as being asked to do something he had no capacity for. I also kept the dialogue concrete, clarifying events, interactions, and feelings.

THE DEFICIT IN A GOOD CONTAINING OBJECT

Edward's lifelong impoverishment of object relations suggested that he lacked the experience of a good containing object. Bion (1962) described how the infant utilizes projective identification to rid itself of overwhelming, disruptive feelings. The mothering figure serves as a container through her reverie, thereby metabolizing the feelings that then become manageable for the infant. Fairbairn (1941) believed that the infant may retain psychic contents because of a fear of loss. Self-expression is experienced as expulsion of the internal object. Evacuation may not only be an expression of the wish to be rid of the object but also an indication to give. Fairbairn did not clarify or explain this suggestive thought. Bringing together Bion's and Fairbairn's ideas, I suggest that internal contents can be given and are not lost only if there is a good containing object to give them to. Abraham (1924) stated that the retention of contents reflects the struggle to retain the internal object in spite of aggression and tenuous object constancy. It would therefore be foolhardy to interpret resistance and elicit aggression. Instead, I focused on the deficit of a good containing object. Edward often remarked that he feared he had nothing to say because he was empty-headed.

Therapist: It's my sense that it's not that you are empty-headed.

Edward: (laughing) I'm afraid maybe there is nothing there. Hollow. No feelings, no thoughts, no ideas.

Therapist: That you are lacking.

Edward: In every way.

Therapist: I think it is important to look precisely at what is lacking. In our sessions with a little help you have had something to say about yourself, your life, and other people.

Edward: That's true.

Therapist: Therefore, it's my sense that it isn't that there isn't anything there, but rather that you are afraid of losing what is there, so you withhold self-expression.

Edward: What do you mean? Losing what is there?

Therapist: That thoughts and feelings are kept from your awareness or consciousness, so you are not needing to express them.

Here I spoke to Edward in the mode of self as object. I did not say, "You keep thoughts and feelings from consciousness," because it was too removed from his experience of being the object of his thoughts and feelings.

Edward: So you are saying it is not just that I am hollow or superficial. Is there a reason for this?

Therapist: There is something I have in mind. When someone tells another person about an important experience or feeling or idea and the other person does not listen, misunderstands, or does not care, it can feel as if whatever was expressed is lost, disappears into a vacuum. The other person does not recognize it as important—it loses its value and becomes meaningless.

Edward: Are there people who actually like to communicate? (laughs)

Therapist: Let's think about it. If the other person values what is said, takes it in, considers it, then gives feedback, it is not lost. Rather, it is returned with a dividend. What is given is returned—with a bonus—what the other puts into it. The recognition.

Here again, I was careful not to discuss Edward as a subject intentionally acting. Rather, I described the experience in terms of what was done to him or how it would be experienced by him.

Edward became aware that he did not retain our discussions.

The inability to remember was another indication of the deficit of a containing object. Not until he had a sense that the therapist valued and retained what he said would Edward begin to hold onto what he said.

> *Edward*: Where are we? I do not recall what was said last time.
> *Therapist*: Maybe if you think about it. (silence) Do you recall?
> *Edward*: Let's see. It's a blank.
> *Therapist*: What made you think of it? Was what you were thinking of related to it?

After allowing some time to see if he remembered, I mentioned one issue we had discussed to stimulate his evocative memory. I mentioned something rather innocuous to provide him with an opportunity to recall what was significant. This usually resulted in his recalling the session. He expressed wonder that I had remembered. My aim was to provide him with the experience of a containing object so that he could identify with this function and begin to value and contain his own inner contents.

The above interventions illustrated the limitations of Edward's caregivers by describing what was omitted in his development—the provision of the containing function. According to Margaret Little (1991), Winnicott termed this holding technique *revelation*. The interpretation does not uncover conflict but rather addresses deficits in parenting that result in deficiency of ego functioning. George Frank (personal communication, September 1980) has pointed out that the patient cannot exercise weak or nonexistent ego functions unless he is aware that they are missing.

THE RECOGNITION OF FAILURES IN CONTAINING

Edward reported that he had been avoiding human contact lately. He did not return phone calls or letters and was avoiding people at work. I explored this further and learned that he usually received negative input from people.

> *Edward*: Bill, the friend I've mentioned, left me a hundred messages. (laughs) I'm exaggerating.
> *Therapist*: Tell me about Bill and your relationship.

Discussing their friendship, he made passing mention that Bill often offered unsolicited advice. When I brought this dissatisfaction to his attention, Edward said the person whose letter he did not answer was always highly critical and ended the letter with an admonishment. Edward added that during this week he had been depleted working overtime every night. He called his sister and in passing complained about how tired he was. She said, "Well, you're getting paid, right?"

Ordinarily, such a remark would not have disturbed him. He was now aware of wanting some empathic recognition, for instance, if she had simply said, "That stinks. You must be tired."

Edward now realized that when he was growing up, no one was permitted to complain: "My parents made you feel that you were an emotional weakling if you asked them for anything."

HOLDING AND THE EMERGENCE OF THE TRUE SELF

Edward began to have a need for contact as a result of the revelation of the omission of good object relationships. He contacted neighbors, persons at work, and friends. He called an old friend, Seth, who invited him to visit for a weekend in the country. Edward was feeling lonely, with little to do in his spare time. He wished to visit Seth but felt it would not be constructive.

> *Therapist*: Constructive?
> *Edward*: Well, Seth is childlike. He never assumes responsibility. He plays all the time. If I go, we will play with the computer, drink beer, play ball, watch games. It will be like two children.

Edward felt that he should be more mature, force himself to go to a museum, read about art, meet new and mature people. His former therapist had encouraged him to face the social situations he feared. I asked him how this had worked out. He said he had tried but had not felt true to himself and had not become more sociable. I remarked that just as Seth was always a child, Edward played at being an adult and never let himself feel childlike. His effort at assuming the role of an adult felt false because he denied the need to play. There was a difference between letting go of responsibilities for a weekend and doing so permanently. I suggested that he consider which activity he really wanted to do—learning about art, going to a museum, and meeting new people could certainly be enjoyable in itself, but so could visiting with a friend and playing.

As Edward felt the need for increased human contacts, his antilibidinal identification with the rejecting parent was activated. He rejected his own need for contact and admonished himself to act maturely. I did not yet interpret this but instead provided a holding explanation that alluded to the true and false self, the positive value of play, and emphasized that he was allowed to make a choice based on his own needs.

THINGS REPLACE PEOPLE

In subsequent sessions, Edward expressed interest in understanding the problems in his past relationships with women. He became aware that he had trouble not only accepting empathy, but also giving to the other. He had always been generous with his time, help, and money, but he lacked the capacity for emotional concern. He described the women throughout his life with little differentiation between them. The breaking off of the relationship with his first wife was revealing of his conflicts around intimacy. As the relationship ended, he had no feelings of sadness, anger, or loss, but only felt concerned about spending and losing all his money even though there was no realistic reason for such concern.

> *Therapist*: Could there be any connection about your anxieties over losing all your money and the loss of the relationship?
> *Edward*: The relationship ending may have made me feel inse-cure and I put this anxiety onto money.
> *Therapist*: You said that there was no realistic reason to be so worried about finances. You cooperated on the settlement, and there was no unsatisfactory change in job or salary, true?

Edward: I was doing well. I just did not feel I was.

Therapist: Is it possible that you placed all of your anxiety on money because you had more control of it than you did over the relationship?

Edward: I think you have something there. I have always been a collector. I like to own things. I have always cared for things more than people. My second wife kidded that I loved my computer more than her. Later it was no longer a joke.

THE SCHIZOID SENSE OF FEELING AS SOLID AS A ROCK

Sartre (1943) said that the self, lacking recognition, experiences a sense of emptiness. The subject seeks to fill the lack by the acquisition of possessions. Acquisition is a way to feel substantial. Taken to the extreme, the sense of substantiality negates lack but results in the subject feeling like a thing in itself, impenetrable, as solid as a rock but without spontaneity, desire, or aliveness. Fairbairn (1940) described phenomenological emptiness in terms of the infant lacking love or recognition from the caregiver. There is an acquisition of internal objects to fill the void. Feces are readily symbolic of the acquired objects. Things in the external world can symbolize feces. Bowlby (1958) described how children exposed to traumatic separation anxiety substitute possession of nonhuman things for human relations. What Bowlby describes in terms of the conscious, observational experience of mother–infant, Fairbairn depicts in the dimension of phantasy and Sartre in terms of phenomenology. Edward responded to disappointments in human relationships by fortifying himself with possessions. However, he then did not feel fully human, but rather like a thing in itself. At this point, he remarked that he experienced himself as without emotions, thoughtlessly satisfied, solid as a rock.

BREAKING UP OF THE INTERNAL OBJECT RELATIONSHIP

Edward recalled that when his first wife left him and they kissed goodbye, he looked over her shoulder at the apartment, thinking it was urgently in need of repair. He had no feelings about the breakup with his wife. He worked furiously on the apartment for several weeks. He realized that he worked compulsively. He was so exhausted that he nearly collapsed.

> *Therapist*: You experienced the loss of your marital relationship through the feeling that your apartment was broken up and in need of repair. The apartment symbolized the broken relationship inside of you. The urgent need to repair the apartment reflects the need to repair the inner broken relationship.

THE UNCONSCIOUS SYMBOL

Wright (1991b) points out that unconscious symbols manifested in dreams are lived through acting and doing in a physical mode. Edward was driven by his need to repair the apartment. Wright says that a metaphor, a higher level of symbolization, is a communication that the subject imagines or uses to express a sensed and nearly discerned hidden aspect of self. Edward's repairing of the apartment was not a metaphor but rather an unconscious symbol. There was a physicality in his compulsivity. Wright explains that through the unconscious symbol, one lives and suffers a psychological situation.

THE EMERGING FEAR OF REJECTION

I took my vacation while treating Edward after only a few months. He had no reaction to the break. He said that everyone needs a vacation. When I returned, he acknowledged being less connected. It felt like beginning over again. Before the vacation, he had begun to think of what we discussed for a day or two after our session. This was a new experience, in that he had never recalled what had been discussed in his previous therapy. Now that I returned, he reverted back to that state. I interpreted that he may have been angry at me for going away and therefore evacuated me from his mind. This interpretation was probably premature, in that he had

no reaction. It was more useful when I provided a holding revelation of the deficit: "You are not accustomed to getting anything of
value from people. It is not surprising that you can't hold onto
feelings about relationships."

I made several similar interventions and he began to think of
what we discussed as he had before. He thought of calling a female
neighbor, Anne. She was mature, accepting, and caring. Their
relationship was not romantic in that Anne had a steady boyfriend.
He could not bring himself to call. When he considered doing so,
the mood left him. He suddenly felt lethargic. I pointed out that this
mood came over him when he wanted to call, so something within
him may have created the mood to prevent the calling. He now
recalled that as he deliberated about calling Anne, he remembered
our previous session. I had said that he feared expressing feelings to
people because he felt they'd reject him. However, he experienced
the thoughts of calling Anne and those about our session as going
along two separate tracks. He realized he did not put together the
simple idea that he hesitated to call Anne because he feared rejection.
He called Anne and she said she was busy that night but could see
him the next day. It was unusual for Edward to take the initiative.
When he got together with people, it was almost always at their
initiative. Only after the call did he realize that he hesitated to call
because of the fear of rejection.

Bion (1967) described the schizoid patient's attacks on linking
in their thought processes. The patient attacks cause-and-effect and
other associative phenomena. The schizophrenic patient suffers
overwhelming envy over dependence on the breast. Therefore,
sadistic attacks on links deny dependence. Edward, an obsessive-
compulsive neurotic with an underlying schizoid core, was not as
severely disturbed as the patients described by Bion. Nevertheless,
he displayed attacks on linking. He attacked the connection between the fear of calling Anne and his lethargy, the fear of impoverishment and the loss of his first wife, the breakup of the
relationship and repair of his apartment.

RESISTING BEING FOR THE OTHER

Edward became increasingly aware of what occurred in his object
relationships. There were occasions when he spoke to someone,

considered the discussion ridiculous, then was surprised when the other gave indication of enjoying the contact. He imagined that the other had interacted only because of a sense of obligation. Edward then made himself agreeable so the other would be less put off. He acknowledged that he related to others primarily out of a sense of obligation. I therefore interpreted that his view of the other as relating only out of obligation was colored by his own experience. He realized that this situation replicated his early family history. Whenever he had asked his parents for anything, they had been self-absorbed and had treated him as a bother. They had not rejected his wishes outright, given that it was important for them to live up to their ideal of good parents, but had responded with a sense of obligation.

Over the next few weeks, Edward became more aware of his sense of obligation. However, he seldom acted on it, but rebelled and felt guilty. If people left messages on his answering machine, he did not respond.

> *Edward*: I feel no wish for contact. There is nothing in it for me.
>
> *Therapist*: There has been no history of good and caring relationships. Is it that you can't imagine them to be pleasurable—to give you something?
>
> *Edward*: I feel strained with people. I am always going along with what they want or think.
>
> *Therapist*: They are strained because you deny yourself the pleasure of self-expression. It is understandable that you don't enjoy being with others because all you have ever known is being for others and accommodating to what they expect.

In our next session Edward said he remained withdrawn and felt he had nothing to give. He felt lonely but did not make contact. I said that his phrase that he had "nothing to give" assumed that the other wanted something. I said, "Your idea of the other person is that he demands, and therefore relating is giving yourself over."

He became more animated than usual in response and recalled various ways he had had to be helpful and to give himself over to his parents throughout childhood. Edward then described how, when people called, he not only felt burdened but also angry, thinking they should leave him be. I remarked that the theme was of being intruded upon. I explored this issue, but he said it was not on the correct track. He said that his parents had not been intrusive, but had wanted to be left alone. In exploring being left alone, he described how he and his brother had shared a large room.

> *Therapist*: How old were you?
> *Edward*: Always. From after I was born. It was strange. My parents were not poor. It was the idea that we should not be in our parents' hair. We were very independent. We played games by ourselves for hours. My mother always boasted about how we could be left alone because we entertained ourselves. It was not that we were deprived. At least, not in the usual way. There were a million things to play with and to do. There was also a tutor—a helper who organized our activities. It was all very structured. The adults set the stage, and we took our cues and carried on exactly as expected.

Winnicott (1971a) described how some children may be overly patterned by their environment. They become precociously independent as they fit into a predetermined patterning of experience. I explained to Edward that his overly accommodating behavior appeared to be based on a lifelong experience of accommodating to an overly patterned familial situation in which he had little opportunity to express his own needs.

INTERPRETING THE PROJECTIVE IDENTIFICATION OF OBJECT RELATIONAL NEEDS

During the first year of treatment, my interventions provided holding revelations of the deficits in Edward's environment that resulted in impaired object relations. He gave indication that it was timely to provide interpretations as internal conflict became manifest in the transference. Edward described a party at work during which his colleagues asked why he never visited them. As he laughed about their efforts, I sensed that he enjoyed the fact that they were frustrated.

Edward: What should I do? Should I force myself to be more sociable? Maybe I will eventually become spontaneously motivated after I receive positive reinforcement for my efforts. My previous therapist always encouraged me to force myself to socialize for those reasons.

Therapist: Did you try this?

Edward: Yes.

Therapist: How did it work?

Edward: It didn't.

Therapist: You are putting into me that part of yourself that wants human contact by wanting me to encourage you to socialize. I am not saying that this is purposeful. You always describe how your friends or colleagues want you to be sociable. When you don't reply to calls or letters, you may be creating concern in them. They then want you to be more social. You then don't have to want to be social for yourself. You reject their efforts, which is the way you reject your own need for contact.

I did not actually make this interpretation at once. Different instances when he described his friends as frustrated and pressuring him to be more related or when he attempted to induce me into this position provided repeated opportunity for interpretation. He became curious about his tendency to reject his own need for contact. He did not yet feel this to be true. He only felt uninterested in contact. Nevertheless, such interpretation of projective identification awakened his curiosity.

INTERPRETING THE REPRESSED LIBIDINAL EGO

Fairbairn (1941) explained that in cases where the neurotic defense successfully covers over the schizoid conflict, the patient is unaware of the unconscious antidependent sadistic rejection of libidinal dependency needs. Therefore, the therapist must continually interpret evidence in the clinical material so that the patient becomes aware of the underlying conflict. My opening interpretation only provided a framework for the working-through process.

Edward witnessed a fight between a shopper and a storekeeper. He was put off by the shopper's show of anger and demand for attention. He recognized that his own anger at the shopper was unjustified and out of proportion to the situation. I remarked that the shopper may represent the dependent childlike self that wants attention and demands to correct grievances. The rage he felt toward the shopper might reflect the rage he felt toward the needy side of himself. He replied that my remarks made sense, but he did not feel that way. Nevertheless, he was interested. There were instances in which he recalled feeling angry at needy ex-girlfriends. I remarked that the girlfriend may represent the mother of his childhood who demanded his help but didn't nurture him. He said he never asked his mother for anything now. In fact, she recently called and asked why he never called or visited. I said he might have avenged himself upon her for rejecting his need for primary love. He did so by communicating, "If you will not give me what I want, then I will not need anything. I reject you as you reject me."

In this way, he rejected his mother but also his own dependency on her. The sadism he felt at seeing friends or colleagues frustrated by his antisocial attitude reflected the phantasy of turning the tables on his mother for rejecting him. One day, he brought in clinical material that provided convincing confirmation of his conflicts. He had visited friends who had a baby. When the baby began to cry and demand, he felt angry. He thought the baby should be stomped on. He also felt angry at the mother for being so tolerant of the baby crying. He thought of the mother as spoiling the baby, exciting its dependence, and creating an insatiable monster. He acknowledged knowing very little about their relationship and that his response had therefore to do with his own inner issues. His anger reflected the antilibidinal ego sadistically rejecting the libidinal ego's need for the exciting mother. I remarked that this situation of an angry, rejecting attitude toward a crying baby's need for a mother was going on inside him all the time. It was usually out of his awareness unless an unavoidable external situation triggered the feelings associated with the conflict. I added that the repression of this conflict permitted him to remain in contact with the world in a cool, distant fashion. If he allowed the conflict expression, it would disturb the minimal contact he had with the outer world. He thought about this and said, "So I withdraw in order to stay in contact."

The next week Edward came in, saying that his life is like sugar-free, fat-free yogurt.

> *Therapist*: What is that like?
> *Edward*: As food, it's great for the body. But it's not good if your life is that way. Kind of pure, ideal but plain, without any passion or zest. My relationships are superficial, sterile. I understood last week that this is how I live emotionally. Very bland.

In the sessions that followed, Edward became angry over a series of incidents in which others did not take his feelings seriously. It was apparent that the frustrated and angry dependent self was beginning to emerge for the first time. It became manifested in the transference situation.

> *Edward*: There is something on my mind—it's ridiculous.
> *Therapist*: Ridiculous?
> *Edward*: Well, infantile—that is what bothers me. It's what you said. This infantile self that I repress to have smooth relationships is coming out here. I sometimes become angry if I lose a minute of a session. Literally a minute. Sometimes you come to me a minute late when you're with another patient. I get upset that I might not get my full time. You might stop right on the dot. It's ridiculous because I literally mean one minute.
> *Therapist*: It is your time and you're entitled to all of it. It's understandable that you don't want to be gypped out of a minute.

THE EMERGENCE OF DEPRESSIVE CONFLICT

Edward began to question about his giving mode of relating. He thought there may be truth to the complaints of the former women in his life that he gave materially but not emotionally. He raised this concern because he had begun to date a new woman whom he liked and did not want to harm the prospect of a relationship.

Fairbairn (1941) suggested that giving is the mature mode of object relating. Originally, the infant relates by taking, but later it is inclined to give or to give back. There is an evolutionary basis to this development, in that mutual cooperation and reciprocity of giving supports the survival of the species. Therefore, I initially emphasized the adaptive aspect of Edward's giving by stating, "The fact that you can give is a strength—it shows concern and is your way of connecting. But let's see if there is a problematic side to it." Through exploration, Edward realized that he sometimes provided help when the other did not need it. I interpreted that Edward's giving seemed related not only to his caring but also to his feelings of insecurity.

In the earlier part of the treatment, Edward's giving behavior was understood as a manifestation of his false-self accommodation toward the object he obliged. There was now a depressive aspect present. Ogden (1986) described the depressive position as a mode of organizing experience relating to omnipotently controlling the object to deny separation, aggression, and guilt. As Edward improved, the theme of loss emerged. Edward's new girlfriend planned an airplane trip. She did not have much money. There was some discussion of Edward paying for her trip. She was ambivalent about taking his help. In the past, he would have taken over the entire trip, planning for it and paying for it. He was now reluctant to do so; they discussed this issue further and she said she was more comfortable paying her own way. For the first time, he experienced separation anxiety, worrying she might meet a man on the trip. Edward now realized that by taking over the trip, he attempted to control her so that he didn't have to risk the possibility of losing her.

Edward now recalled that he was told that when he was 6 months old, his parents had taken a vacation to Latin America for several weeks. He had always been told that he was a good baby and did not protest. Although he could not remember the incident, he became angry and saddened that his parents were so detached as to leave him at such a vulnerable time. He felt that if they had been excited about caring for him, they would not have left. He connected his lifelong need to accommodate and give to others as a reaction to the early loss.

Bowlby (1958) described infants suffering from premature traumatic object loss as giving up on their dependence on the parental objects and turning to compulsive possession of non-human objects or taking care of human objects. Edward showed both of these reactions in his efforts to compensate for early object loss.

As he began to be aware of the issues of object loss, he became pained and frustrated by the intervals between sessions. I suggested that he may be reliving the frustration and pain of waiting for the return of his parents. At this point, he recalled instances of waiting for his mother terrified that she would never return. He detached himself when she did return so as to protect himself.

As he struggled with these depressive themes, he felt deeply about the unhappiness of his second wife. He felt that she had been serious about wishing to have a close and meaningful life with him but that he did not have the capacity to love. When she became ill and died, he detached himself. He now mourned the loss of his second wife. He was preoccupied with fantasies of reparation in which he now communicated to her his understanding of her pain and loss. There was increased separateness as he experienced longing and sadness that he never could in reality communicate to her. The mourning of the second wife was also a reliving of the early loss of his mother.

For the first time Edward reported a need to tell others about feelings of loss. He had told his sister, a friend, and his girlfriend. This was definitely a new feeling—to release painful emotions. The stress in his life affected him physically. His stomach was upset and he suffered from diarrhea. He also felt mildly depressed for the first time. He described diarrhea as getting rid of the junk he ate. I pointed out that he was also feeling a need to get rid of troubling emotions. I reminded him of our earlier discussions of his need to hold onto painful emotions—precious contents he feared losing—that self-expression was felt as a loss because there was no one to receive and to value them. I said that now his ridding himself of these emotions about people was a form of separation and loss and caused him to feel depressed. I added that at the same time, he is not simply losing his feelings because there is now the idea of sharing them with others since he wants to express his feelings to different persons.

Edward wondered if he was just dumping his feelings onto others. He said he did not want anything back from them, nor was he especially interested in what they had to say. He read in a popular

magazine about people who narcissistically unloaded feelings. Although he never before heard the phrase, it resonated with how he
felt about expressing his feelings to other people. I agreed that he
had not yet reached the capacity for reciprocity. He could not yet
think of a give-and-take or find value in what the other person had
to say in response to himself. At the same time, there was an
important change because he not only wanted to rid himself of
feelings but wished to talk about them to another person. Therefore, giving to another was involved. I then asked if there was a
reason he selected the particular people he chose to talk to. He said
that all of them listened sympathetically. I pointed out there was a
change— that he had the idea of a caring listener to whom he could
give his inner contents. The feelings could be expressed without
being lost. I said there was still some feeling of loss because there
was now the idea of another to contain the feelings for safekeeping
but there was not yet the idea of the other giving back meaningful
feedback—a return of what was given but transformed by the
other.

SPLITTING IN THE TRANSFERENCE

Edward manifested splitting in the transference. He reported that
on his way to the session, he passed a nearby hospital and thought
about the poor medical care in the city. There was a man standing
outside the hospital looking forlorn and lost. Edward imagined that
he was a patient in need of help. He wondered if the man was ill or
homeless and waiting for medical treatment. Edward felt relieved
that he was not in the man's place. Earlier in the week, during his
lunch break, he went to an HMO clinic for a checkup. He expected
to be in and out quickly. The waiting room was filled with persons
he imagined to be on welfare, or to be mentally ill or taken care of
by the government. He was annoyed at having to wait. He thought
that the system and such bureaucracies as the clinic providing care
for the indigent and needy maintained them in a dependent, helpless
position. He imagined that the clinic provided unnecessary tests and

was part of a bureaucratic system that excited endless need by doling out welfare, Medicaid, and so forth. He said that the helpers did not really care. Furthermore, the clinic staff probably did not consider a middle-class patient like himself important when there were so many needy people. He did not believe the staff cared more about them, but rather that they were so overwhelmed by their overwhelming needs that they did not have the time or energy to pay attention to him.

I remarked that he was complaining about poor treatment and not receiving proper attention because the physician was over-whelmed by needier patients. I pointed out that he also came for treatment and wondered if he felt this way about the therapy. He said that his feelings about the therapy were not at all the same as his feelings about the clinic or hospital. He felt that I paid attention and was not overwhelmed, but he admitted that he wondered if I would not take his statements the wrong way. I raised the possibility that the needy patients could stand for the dependent side of himself, whereas I could stand for the bureaucratic, overwhelmed physician or system that excites but does not meet his needs. He felt no awareness of this state and instead believed his attitude to our relationship to be entirely rational and professional. I agreed that it was, but I reminded him that in his story he was rejecting toward the needy patients and the system and said it was possible that he similarly rejected those feelings in his relationship to me and that this was why he had no awareness of them. This idea interested him and he laughed, saying, "So then it would be like I have two relationships to you—the cooperative one I am aware of and the other in which I am dependent and frustrated." I said that would be correct and that he rejected the dependent, frustrated aspect. He said that our cooperative relationship did not feel false. He felt that he was involved, trying to understand himself, and that the therapy was helpful. He admitted that this description was rather ideal. I acknowledged that his cooperative attitude was not false and that he did try hard to understand himself, which is the aim of therapy. I added that, since the therapy was actually working in that way and he found it to be helpful, he would feel irrational if he allowed for the dependent, frustrated feelings that he likened to the needy patients. Given that he did not in reality experience an uncaring or overwhelmed bureaucrat, if he became aware of such transferential feelings, he would have to look for their source.

He understood these remarks and said when he awakened that morning he thought that he had nothing to discuss in therapy today. Walking to his session, he thought about his first wife. He remembered the ways that they had disappointed and frustrated each other. He became angry. It was at this point that he passed the hospital, saw the forlorn patient, and recalled the visit to the HMO clinic. I remarked that the unconscious is nearest expression upon awakening because dreaming is the state where it reigns. I said it was possible that his thought about having nothing to say today may have been an unconscious command not to think or say anything. Thinking about his first wife, the hospital, and the clinic may have all indicated that the needy, dependent self was demanding expression. That could disrupt his cooperative, ideal relationship to me. If it could be kept down, unheard and unfelt, he could continue to receive the ideal treatment without it getting in the way. Since he and his first wife often provoked one another, and institutions did in reality often provide inadequate care, these situations lent themselves to displacing the unacceptable transferential feelings.

He now thought about the origin of the disruptive, split-off transferential feelings. He realized that his family life, in many ways, had been a bureaucracy. He and his siblings had been provided with numerous "things," their activities had always been patterned and structured, yet they had been shown little care or affection. I remarked that he grew up repressing the dissatisfaction and anger over this state of affairs to get along in the world. Therapy, being a helping relationship, often awakens unmet early needs. The object of such needs had been a bureaucraticlike family that did not respond adequately. When the object of one's needs feels exciting, frustrating, rejecting, and bad, the needs themselves are experienced that way. The entire situation is repressed—needs, objects, and all. I said that the resulting relationship to the world is not so disruptive but lacks feeling. Edward replied that his world felt like sugar-free, fat-free, cholesterol-free yogurt because he had rejected not only the frustrating object of his needs, but also the needs themselves.

Fairbairn (1943) stated that libido is experienced as "bad" and therefore rejected because the object the libido is attached to is felt to be bad, that is, exciting but frustrating or rejecting. Libido is thus unavailable for external object relations, lessening the patient's capacity for meaningful, emotional connection. The result is an ideal but superficial relationship to the external object world.

WITHDRAWAL AND COMPETITION

Toward the end of the second year of treatment, I took vacation. Edward went to visit with old friends around the same time. He reported that his friends were extremely competitive. They competed with talking, debating, and playing golf, basketball, and Frisbee. Whenever he saw them, their entire time together was spent in such competition. In the past, he always stood aside, somewhat withdrawn. They all talked, not allowing each other to get in a word edgewise. There was an oral quality, as if a group of children were grabbing at urgently needed food. For the first time, he insisted on his say and did not stand on the side. When they played ball, he also did his best. In the past, he had always felt passive, week, and tired. Now he had energy and aggression.

He had grown up with those friends. His way of relating to them, he now realized, replicated his way in his family. He allowed his siblings and parents to take center stage. His younger brother and father were highly aggressive and competitive, reminding him of his friends. His sister and mother were demanding and needy, reminding him of his first wife. In the family he stepped aside as everyone fought and noisily competed for needed supplies. He recalled being on a train and seeing several youths who, he imagined, lived in the suburbs and visited the city. All but one boy were lively and loud, laughing and kidding. The one youth stood to the side, dressed in the same casual clothes as the others, looking in appearance as if he fit in but withdrawn, not enthusiastically taking

part in the horsing around. He was like this youth—part of the
group, yet not completely. A part of him was there, but a deeper
part was not fully present, and was unnoticeable to the others.

Guntrip (1969) stated that impingement and neglect were
most likely to result in the regressed, passive ego, while overstimulation and overt rejection were likely to result in the active oral
sadomasochistic libidinal ego. Edward suffered primarily from
early neglect and impingement, giving rise to the regressed and
withdrawn libidinal ego. I first interpreted the splitting off of the
active libidinal ego and the exciting object in the transference as
revealed in the fantasy of ill treatment by the medical bureaucracy.
The needy and demanding patients Edward envied and hated represented not only his active oral libidinal self but also his siblings,
whom he had stepped aside for in his withdrawn state. He projected
his active oral libidinal self onto his siblings and competitive peers
while he retreated into the withdrawn, regressed state. As he no
longer expressed the active libidinal ego, he emerged from his
withdrawn state.

13

INTEGRATING THE FRAGMENTED EGO

Elizabeth is a female patient in her mid-thirties. An executive, she lives independently and has been in twice-weekly treatment for four years. Like Edward, Elizabeth suffers from an obsessive-compulsive neurosis defending against a schizoid core. However, unlike Edward, Elizabeth loses the internal object under stress and sometimes suffers the actual schizoid state. It will be recalled that Edward did not risk losing the internal object until he had a good enough internal containing object to give it over to. Unable to hold onto the internal object, Elizabeth loses it without a containing object to give it over to. It is this situation that results in the actual schizoid experience. The therapist must therefore serve more as a holding object in management of the therapeutic regression. Whereas the case of Edward illustrated a predominance of interpretive intervention, Elizabeth's demonstrates holding and management for a patient with similar dynamics.

PERSONAL HISTORY

Elizabeth grew up in an intact family with an older brother. She described her mother as domineering and intrusive but emotionally

distant and exceedingly uncomfortable with physical contact. She
described her father as passive and emotionally absent. Her mother
was overbearing about wanting to know Elizabeth's whereabouts,
the friends she was with, or what she did at school. There was a
feeling of not being able to get out of her mother's sight. Her
mother would say, "I always know what you're up to—even when
you're not here—and what I don't know God knows. Remember,
He is always watching—you are never alone." At times Elizabeth
felt comforted and protected by the idea of the hovering presence of
her mother and God. As she grew older, however, she increasingly
felt spied upon. In adolescence, she admiringly stared at her developing body in the mirror, then imagined God watching her
watching herself and covered up in shame. She fantasized that she
could be out of God's sight for limited periods by breathing rapidly
four times in succession. She then became obsessively concerned
that she had miscounted or that she needed to renew the count,
imagining the intrusive return of God's eye. There were other
occasions when she doubted the existence of God and her parents
seemed to be old and ignorant with foolish beliefs. She then felt
isolated, frightened, as if she were not real. She longed for God even
though the idea oppressed her.

Elizabeth described her father as well meaning but ineffectual.
He had a history of major depression and was withdrawn from the
family life. He was a brilliant man but never lived up to his
potential. Elizabeth's older brother, Fred, was dependent on their
mother and suffered from volatile mood swings and a violent
temper. Elizabeth felt that her mother overprotected him and over-
looked his destructive behavior. During their childhood, he often
took her belongings or intruded on her. She complained, but her
parents did not confront him and instead told her to overlook it.
When she became angry or fought with him, her parents usually
sided with her brother, saying it was her fault because she was not
emotionally disturbed and so should know better. Her brother
demanded a great deal from their parents, while Elizabeth stoically
drew on her own resources. She was an agreeable, quiet child but
not overly compliant. Her brother complained that she was favored
because she was the youngest, received excellent grades in school,
and was rewarded for her hard work. In the evening, her mother

went to the rooms of both children for a goodnight talk. She went to see Fred first, spending much time discussing his problems. By the time she came to Elizabeth, she was exhausted. Elizabeth allowed her to spend less time. Her mother also avoided kissing her goodnight. Elizabeth occasionally insisted and felt her mother's discomfort.

Elizabeth was a good student academically but did not easily make friends or become involved in after-school activities. She did have one best girlfriend. The two were inseparable and confided in one another about everything. She believed that she and her friend had been considered studious nerds by the more popular high school students. They were made fun of, but not to the point of being scapegoated. Elizabeth was awkward in appearance and not very confident. Her friend, Margaret, was attractive physically and, although not very popular, was self-assured and stylishly dressed. Elizabeth admired her and felt complimented that Margaret had selected her as a best friend. A third girl joined their friendship for one summer. Margaret became close with the third girl and Elizabeth had felt rejected. The third girl, who was very popular, rejected Margaret upon returning to school. Elizabeth demanded that Margaret admit to mistreating her before resuming their friendship. After they were friends again, Elizabeth could not entirely let go of her anger. Elizabeth went through college and graduate school, performing on a superior level academically. In the first years of both college and graduate school there was a lapse in her usual performance and strained relations with peers.

DIFFICULTIES WITH INTIMACY

Elizabeth sought therapy because of a lack of intimate relationships in her adult life. She had never been involved in a long-lasting relationship with a man, nor had she been sexually involved. She had experienced brief infatuations that had not developed into relationships. She had male and female friends with whom she socialized occasionally. However, she usually stayed alone in her apartment on weekends. She spent hours going through the newspaper, watching television talk shows or movies on the VCR. These activities were not problems in themselves, but she felt that there was a passive, withdrawn quality to it. She planned to be active, to call friends, or to go out, but she became absorbed in these activities for too prolonged a time and could not get herself moving. By the end of the weekend she felt that she had wasted her time. She also reported symptoms of feeling an urgent need to urinate and sometimes to defecate when she was in a claustrophobic situation. The symptoms came over her in business meetings, on dates, or on airplanes directly after it was announced that people could not leave their seats during take-off or landing. She checked out the problem medically and no physiological problem was found. She also complained of feeling stuck in her corporate position. She earned an excellent salary and was valued by the firm. She worked in a department where she did not have one supervisor but worked on several projects for different persons. This department was considered the starting point, and employees were typically promoted to other departments. She feared any change, although her employers were hinting it was time.

Elizabeth was fastidiously dressed. She wore tailored business suits and never had a hair out of place. She gave an impression of looking very put together, an appearance that belied her internal state, which she described as falling apart.

THE DYADIC STATE

In our first session Elizabeth described a dream in which she was stood up by a man. I asked what she made of it and she said that she did not have any dates recently so that it must be about how her relationships didn't work out. I pointed out that it was her dream and that she unconsciously created the narration and produced it so that she was stood up and disappointed. She replied that her relationships often turned out that way—the other person disappointed her.

> *Therapist*: Then it would be all the more reason for your unconscious dream teller to have this story work out differently— that you got what you wished for—a dream does not have to follow

the circumstances of your life. Especially if they're unhappy. But your dream is in accord with the very state of affairs you wish to change—you don't even change them in a dream where you can do as you wish. What do you make of that?

Elizabeth: So the dream follows the story of my life. You're saying that I could have dreamed my dream differently than I live my life but didn't.

Therapist: I'm not saying this is purposeful. It isn't that you say, "Let's have this bad dream tonight." But an unconscious part of you narrates the dream and has it turn out a certain way, and this part of you is having it turn out exactly like your life circumstances. It's similar to a person in a prison dreaming he's in prison instead of dreaming he's free.

Elizabeth experienced herself as lived by her life. Like the dream, she experienced relationships as not working out for her. She feels stood up, abandoned, disappointed. She has no sense of herself as a subject contributing to what happens. Wright (1991d) has pointed out that the infant experiences itself as lived by the symbiotic union with the mother. The infant at first cannot psychically stand outside the relationship to the caregiver and see itself in interaction with the mother—both creating and responding to the object. The adult patient primarily experiencing dyadic object relations is enmeshed with internal objects projected onto external relationships. The patient feels lived by her circumstances, an object of experience living in the impulse or need that is excited or rejected by the object. My interpretation is aimed at illustrating to Elizabeth that she is not lived by her dream but creates the dream. Thus I am here performing a paternal function by inviting her to view herself in the dream from the outside, from my perspective. In *Critique of Dialectical Reason* Sartre (1960) described how the unity of a dyad, the contributing of both partners, can only be realized in a totalization performed by an outside third party. The totalization allows for a larger perspective. Thus Elizabeth is not only lived by her dream but lives or creates her dream. This is the first step toward illustrating that she is not only lived by her life but creating or living her life situation. The dream in which she is stood up reflects her life in which she is always unconsciously creating a disappointing situation.

Elizabeth had an obsessional style of speech. She deliberately paused before selecting the perfect word, afraid of saying the wrong thing, of giving the wrong idea. The gap in her speech left the other waiting with nothing, while she was preoccupied with endless possibilities or words she could choose. This obsession suggested that words meant more to her than the meaning of the idea in her mind. Rather, a word was a thing in itself.

My initial interpretations were off the mark. When she described her difficulties in the first years of college and graduate school or her conflicts about job promotion, I interpreted along oedipal lines about avoidance of competition or success. She said these interpretations did not hit home or evoke relevant associations. When she was distressed by a critical, demanding female supervisor, I remarked on the struggle with internal persecutory parental figures to no avail. There was no recognition of significance to these oedipally oriented interpretations.

HUNGER FOR THE OBJECT AND THE LOSS OF AUTONOMY

In the first year of treatment, Elizabeth dated a man who had been introduced by a mutual friend. This relationship lasted for four months, the longest one she had ever had. The man seemed to like her and enjoyed their time together. She responded with overwhelming need that threatened to consume her. Upon exploration, she revealed that she had felt the same way on past occasions and none of those relationships had worked out. She wondered if the intensity of her feelings hadn't driven the others away. She attempted to check the overwhelming feeling of infatuation and not allow it to carry her away since she did not want to ruin this new relationship. I remarked on the urgency of the need, that she hardly knew this man although she had a sense that she liked him. I pointed out that the intensity of the need was out of proportion with what was going on in the relationship. Furthermore, since she had had the same feelings on various other occasions with other men she was getting to know, it did not have to do with any of the particular men but with something within her. It was important to make this intervention repeatedly because the patient entering into this intense dyadic relationship experiences all of her feelings as excited by the object, which in turn creates a greater feeling of enmeshment. I emphasized that the intensity and urgency of the need suggested that it originated long ago and had to do with dependency. I also remarked that much of the time that she described being alone and avoiding relationships may have been a protective maneuver to keep at bay this intense longing. I pointed out that the intense longing may relate to the childhood neglect she had described. I said, "Such childhood neglect created a longing to be recognized and loved, which is also felt to be a threat since it is so urgent and all-consuming."

There were occasions when she came into a session complaining that the new boyfriend might be rejecting her. When we explored the incident carefully, there was sometimes an indication that he had tried to become more involved and that she had become frightened of the closeness and had sought a reason to withdraw. There were also instances when he had actually drawn her close but then had pushed her away.

There is always the question in analytic therapy about how best to address the motivations or conduct of the persons in the patient's life. Patients like Elizabeth with severe difficulties in early object relationships often understand the actions of others in relationship to themselves. If the other is loving, it is because the patient is lovable. If the other is unavailable, it is because the patient is unlovable. Furthermore, the patient relating primarily in a dyadic, symbiotic union cannot accept separateness and understands the object's separate acts as an abandonment. She cannot understand that the object can behave solely in terms of its own needs or wishes separate from the patient. In this situation I pointed out the connection between the closeness and distancing. I then questioned Elizabeth as to what it might mean that the boyfriend called her when she stopped pursuing him but did not call her when she pursued him. If she pursued him and he distanced, she felt it was because she was unlovable. I pointed out that it may be her feeling of being unlovable that caused her to pursue him and that he might distance because of a fear of closeness. This resulted in her feeling even more unlovable and pursuing even more intensely. Elizabeth had enough ego strength to step back from the relationship and perceive it from my totalizing outside perspective. The boyfriend also needed her to adopt his tastes in food, movies, politics, and so forth. At first Elizabeth felt that there was something wrong with her if she thought differently. For a brief period, she went along with his inclinations, but this did not enhance the relationship, since he tended to feel merged in when she was agreeable. She was then able to differentiate herself and realize that he needed her to like what he liked or he felt rejected. His behavior in this regard was quite similar to that of her own mother, who was domineering. By helping her to understand the behavior and possible motivations of the boyfriend and the mother he represented, I offered a holding function of revelation and also a framework for understanding, providing words and meaning to sort out the dyadic interactions.

When the relationship ended after four months, Elizabeth felt a sense of accomplishment. She was not overwhelmed by feelings of infatuation, nor did she blame herself that it did not work out. She felt that both of them had brought difficulties to the relationship, but that she was becoming more aware and could stop herself from acting out.

REGRESSION AND THE BODY

During the second year of her treatment, Elizabeth developed a lower back problem. She typically sat in a chair during our sessions, but with the back strain, she chose to lie on the couch. She also began to come late for sessions. It was my sense that the backache, which was making it difficult for her to get around, reflected a wish for regression, to retreat from the struggle to hold herself together to assume the responsibilities of her life. A physical therapy specialist she went to for treatment told her that the back muscles involved were those that were often used to hold things together when the person was falling apart emotionally or psychically.

LACAN AND THE FRAGMENTED SELF

Jacques Lacan (1949) was the first psychoanalyst to describe the importance of mirroring to the child's developing sense of self. He referred to the child's fascination with its reflected image in the mirror. There is a gap between the child's disjointed and fragmented sense of bodily self, incapable of performing the motoric acts it desires, and the mirrored image of itself as unitary, bounded, and complete. The child then identifies with and internalizes this mirrored image of itself. The infant adopts this complete mirrored image as a character of armor to feel complete. However, this unitary self is false, in the sense that it contradicts its actual state of incompleteness. Thus the mirror image is the child's first objectified sense of self. The child may then exhibit this objectified self to others for mirroring to feel whole and together. However, this sense of completeness contradicts its subjective inner incompleteness. Lacan also described how the bodily self is then experienced as a container for the internal, disjointed, fragmented parts. This bodily container self remains false in that it is identified with the mirror image of the body as complete.

I am not a Lacanian and agree with Winnicott (1971c) that the infant's first mirror is its mother and that the reflection of itself that it later discovers in the mirror is that which its mother has already seen. However, the Lacanian description is quite relevant for an understanding of pathology. Elizabeth's back strain reflected an effort to keep herself together with the threat of an increasing sense of inner fragmentation. Earlier, I discussed how she dressed and groomed herself perfectly to give the appearance of being put together. She then presented this perfect image to the external world for mirroring to belie her internal sense that she could fall apart. At the same time, she never felt authentic or real. She suffered from a pervasive sense of depersonalization that she did not quite fit into her own body. This was coupled by an increasing urgent need to urinate or defecate when feeling closed in. Thus the sense that she was internally disintegrating was reflected in the fear of losing her urine or feces.

DIFFERENTIATING THE SELF FROM THE SELF IMAGE

Around this time, there were important changes in her life to account for the escalation of symptoms. Months after the breakup

of the relationship discussed above, she met a second man considerably more available for a relationship. Elizabeth became involved
with him sexually and, after some initial anxiety, was able to enjoy
physical intimacy. She found being in the relationship stressful.
After a few months, he invited her to spend weekends with him.
Their relationship continued to progress, but she experienced panic
attacks. Upon exploration, she stated, "It is being under scrutiny all
weekend. Being with another person means being observed. I don't
mean he's always watching. It's that being watched is inevitable
when you're with someone day in and day out. I never thought of it
before, but this seems to be the reason I always avoided relationships. I have to keep observing myself to make sure I don't do
anything to spoil the relationship because he's there. This is the
strain. I'm not accustomed to it."

The issue here was one that we discussed for several weeks.
She was observing herself being observed and the question she
always asked was whether her image of herself coincided with his
image of her—and where it did not, who was mistaken. Wright
(1991b) has noted that consciousness is related to sorting out the
image of the object from the object itself and self-consciousness to
sorting out the image of the self from the self as object. Elizabeth's
work in therapy fell into this second area.

The boyfriend had been violently abused and neglected as a
youngster. In his adolescence, he was prone to substance and
alcohol abuse. He had been in psychotherapy for many years, had
given up all drugs and acting out, and had pushed himself hard to
function. Sometimes he could be critical of Elizabeth. For instance,
she was concerned about eating the right food, sleeping enough,
and resting if she had a stressful day at work. He felt this was
self-indulgent behavior. He always pushed himself and didn't pay
attention to what he ate, how much he slept, or whether he was
stressed. Elizabeth had to sort out whether she actually considered
herself to be self-indulgent or whether his judgment was based on
his own issues and not on her. This was a new experience, because
she never had been close enough to anyone to allow him to see her
and describe her. At first, she was unsure if he was correct. We spent
the next session sorting out her self-protective behavior. There was
discussion about how she herself felt that she was sometimes overly

cautious in her self-care. She attributed this to her sense that she could fall apart under stress. She felt the self-care to be realistic because she was not emotionally strong. If she became stronger emotionally, she might need less self-protection. But she also realized that the boyfriend's ideas were based on his own issues. Struggling to change his former acting out tendencies, he sometimes pushed himself unrealistically. She also wondered if his neglect of eating, sleeping, or resting was not a reliving and internalization of the abuse and neglect he suffered as a child. The positive aspect of their relationship was that she could discuss her concerns and what happened between them and he took her seriously. She also pointed out that most of her concerns about feeling under scrutiny were not based on his behavior, in that he was only occasionally critical.

THE SECRET SELF AND THE GAZE OF THE OTHER

Winnicott described both the need of the infant to be mirrored by the mother to feel genuine and alive and the need for an aspect of the infant to remain out of communication, unviolated and protected from impingement. He referred to this second state as the secret self. In a previous publication I (Seinfeld 1991b) described how the need for mirroring and the need for secrecy can be understood in dialectical relationship to one another. Drawing on Sartre's idea that the other's look objectifies and alienates the self, I suggested that the infant initially needs to be mirrored but then inevitably feels captured in the reflection of the mirroring other. Even if the other mirrors the infant for what it is and does not see the infant according to its own needs, or as an extension of it, or doesn't see the infant at all, there is nevertheless a moment of alienation because the infant is being for the other or being what the other sees it to be. Thus, experiencing itself as an object of the other, the infant must annihilate the other's view of it. I would see this critical point, on the part of the infant, as what Wright (1991b) described as the development of self-consciousness in terms of distinguishing itself as an object

from the other's view of it as an object. It is at this point that the
secret self emerges. At this point, the caregiver hopefully responds,
as Winnicott described in *The Capacity to Be Alone* (1958), by
remaining present but permitting the child its solitude. The child,
hiding, unseen, out of sight of the present object, returns to find
itself existing in the eye of the object, only to return again to the
place of hiding. This dialectical process is another way of describing
the separation–reunion occurring throughout separation–individuation. It is when the caregiver does not allow the child the moment of
being alone, but instead attempts to intrude and see the child in its
place of hiding, that the self is disintegrated. Elizabeth felt she was
always in her mother's sight. Later, she felt that God was always
watching. There was no place to escape the spying eye. When she
finally did fantasize an imaginary contract where God would not
see her for an allotted period of time, she felt lost and abandoned.

A difficulty in the treatment of such patients is that the very
aim of the therapy, getting to know and understand the patient, is a
threat to the autonomy and privacy of the secret self. The therapist
therefore must proceed very slowly, seeing only as much as the
patient is ready to reveal. The patient's autonomy is enhanced as she
discovers that the relationship develops without violating her sense
of self.

As she became involved in a relationship, Elizabeth also made
a significant change at work. After much obsessive deliberation, she
accepted a promotion to a new department. This new position
meant that she would be responsible for a single project with a
regular supervisor. Therefore, she was now under scrutiny on the
job as well.

EXPULSION OF THE INTERNAL OBJECT

These changes in relationship and at work resulted in a dramatic
escalation of symptoms. Elizabeth could not sit in a meeting at work
or be in situations with her boyfriend without being overcome by
an urgent need to urinate. The symptoms became so extreme that
she was having difficulty going into work and sometimes took off
half-days or whole days. Her eating and sleeping were both severely affected. She called her boyfriend several times a day. Al-

though he was generally supportive, she felt that she was taxing his patience. I gave her permission to call me whenever she wished and saw her for extra sessions as necessary. During this time, I expressed interest in her somatic as well as her emotional complaints. Wherever appropriate, I referred her to a suitable physician. As Winnicott (1972) pointed out, the psyche and soma are inseparable and the therapist's attention to the patient's somatic complaints, especially during a regressive period, is experienced as holding. Elizabeth said, "I cannot contain myself. Everything is spilling over. I'm flooded by my feelings." Her body was no longer serving her as a container and her insides were experienced as leaking out. As she allowed herself to be scrutinized by the object, she relived the penetrating look of her mother and felt herself to be shattered.

Fairbairn stated that in obsessive-compulsive states, the client experiences the conflict around engulfment versus abandonment in relationship to inner contents of the mind or body. Feeling engulfed by the internal object is experienced as if one is about to explode, a bursting fullness. Separation from the object is experienced as evacuation or expulsion. When Elizabeth felt flooded, that she had to urinate, that she was bursting with anxiety, that she wanted to jump out of her skin, she felt engulfed and needed to evacuate the internal object. The fear of urinating and defecating in public expressed her fear of loss of control, of losing the internal object, and being lost herself. Unlike the patient described in Chapter 12, Elizabeth barely had the strength to retain the internal object; when she temporarily lost it, there was not yet a good enough object to contain it. Thus evacuation was experienced as loss and not giving and thereby resulted in the regressed, schizoid state. The unconscious phantasy of losing internal objects was reflected by a psychic state of fragmentation that impeded her capacity to function. I referred her to a psychopharmacologist for antianxiety medication so that she was not entirely overwhelmed.

MERGER ANXIETY AND EXPULSION OF THE OBJECT

Whenever there was an opportunity, I interpreted the internal object situation. One of Elizabeth's supervisors was a critical, demanding older woman. The supervisor piled up assignments, demanding that they be done in an unreasonably short time. It was in meetings with this person that Elizabeth experienced the urgent need to urinate. I interpreted that she was angry and felt trapped by the demanding supervisor. The urgent need to urinate was the somatic expression of feeling pissed off. I said that urinating expressed her wish to rid herself of the supervisor. She agreed with this interpretation, but she felt that the symptoms were so pervasive and frequent that they did not only apply to anger.

Shortly thereafter, I was provided with an opportunity to make a convincing interpretation of the engulfment-expulsion theme. Elizabeth and her boyfriend were going to a wedding. She dreaded going, fearing she would have to urinate. In the chapel during the wedding, she was seized by a terrible urge to urinate but remained in control until she appropriately found a bathroom afterwards. During our session, she obsessed exclusively about the nature and severity of the symptoms. After a while I stated, "I understand that you suffered a great deal and it is important that you describe this, but it is also important to look at some of the personal problems and issues about relationships that the symptoms are expressing." I was then able to draw her into a discussion of the wedding. It was a close friend who was married, the very friend who introduced her to the boyfriend. At one point during the wedding, Elizabeth wondered if she and her boyfriend would someday marry. However, she was too obsessed by the need to urinate to give this any further thought. I remarked that the interpersonal events that might give rise to anxiety about closeness and separation are denied any significance. However, they trigger anxiety, which is displaced onto bodily concerns. These concerns replace those about relationship. She asked if I could explain this.

> *Therapist*: Going to a chapel, a wedding, for the very person who introduced you and your boyfriend could trigger anxiety about your own relationship. Will there be a commitment? How close are you? Might you even be married someday? This frightens you. There is the need to escape. This is expressed in the need to urinate. The fear of being trapped in this relationship is felt as the feeling that you will burst inside. There is here a wish to piss away the relationship that you fear.

Elizabeth thought of another memory that validated my remark. Several years ago she was attracted to a man in college. To her
surprise, he asked her out. They took a subway to their destination,
but the train became stuck between stations. She suddenly felt an
urgent need to urinate. The thought was in the back of her mind all
along, but the train's being stuck brought it to the fore. She was so
desperate she nearly ran off the subway. Her panic ruined the date.
She realized that she had feared being trapped in the relationship.
The urgent need to urinate reflected the unconscious phantasy of
evacuating the object.

DREAMS REVEALING GREATER INNER AUTONOMY

Elizabeth presented dreams indicating that she was becoming more
autonomous. She dreamed of returning to her parents' home. It was
a group living situation for the elderly. She greeted her parents and
explored the premises. The thought occurred that she could no
longer return home to live because the rooms had been put to other
use. She felt a sense of relief. Shortly afterwards she dreamed of
moving out of her parents' home. She believed this dream was
evidence of growth and separation because she now thought of
leaving of her own free will rather than depending on an external
situation to enforce separation.

Elizabeth gradually grew more comfortable about being in a
love relationship and became less panicked at work. She decided
that she did not like her current job and found a new position that
placed her even more directly under the scrutiny of superiors. The
new job was in another town, which meant she would have to
move. In one dream she was driving, probably through London,
because the traffic was going in the opposite direction. She drove in
the wrong direction or the wrong lane and had to turn to go in the
direction of traffic. She followed some cars off the main road onto a
small, quiet road. She had to come to an abrupt stop because the
road suddenly dropped. It was a dirt road strewn with rocks. She
thought that it was manageable but would be a rough ride. She
awakened.

Elizabeth associated that the dream symbolized her life and therapy. As in the dream, her life and therapy were moving, but she was uncertain of the direction or the end result. As in the dream, she felt she had been going in the wrong direction, one that differed from that of other persons. Now she wanted to go in the same direction so she would not be isolated. She took a turn in her life by starting a new job, having a love relationship, changing residences. She guessed that the steep incline and rocky road meant it would sometimes be rough going and she might not always feel in control. At the same time, it looked manageable. She felt that she stopped before the steep hill to prepare herself for the difficult but, hopefully, manageable road ahead.

THE TRUE AND FALSE SELF AS MANIFEST IN A DREAM

Shortly thereafter, Elizabeth reported a recurring dream that illustrated issues of the true and false self and where they fit into her current level of functioning. She dreamed that someone telephoned. The person asked for Mary. Elizabeth told the caller it was the wrong number. The caller could have been a male or female. The name Mary had no special significance. In other dreams the caller asked for a different name—it might be Bill, Alice, or John. Elizabeth's first association was that she had been called upon to take care of various things. There were issues coming her way that she was called upon to manage—the new job, quitting the old job, her boyfriend going away for a few weeks. Elizabeth wished that it was someone else called upon to handle these things. She felt that the facade she presented when faced with the demands of living was not really her genuine self. She always appeared able and willing but underneath felt overwhelmed and wished to be left alone. She did not wish to work so hard, but the persons she worked with would never know. It was as if someone else—a false part of herself— responded to these demands. She said that the ringing of the phone in the dream was also important. She hated intrusion. If someone is approaching a house, coming by way of the front path, then ringing the doorbell, there is time to prepare. The ringing phone can be the ultimate intrusion in terms of not knowing who or what is coming. Having a caller dial the wrong number was a way of protecting herself from intrusion—the call was for someone else, so she did not have to respond.

I interpreted that the mask or false self—that part of herself always willing to face whatever demands arise—may well have developed in reaction to intrusions, as symbolized by the ringing phone. The demands may also symbolize the demands of early life, forcing her to respond precociously while protecting her true nature from intrusion. It was as if one part of her falsely performed as expected but screened another part of herself that just wished to be left alone. I said, "You often say that when you are partaking in an activity, you do not feel as if all of you participates; that it is as if you are going through the motions but not fully there. This is because there is a part of you that is not participating or involved." Her eyes welled up with tears and she said she was sad at thinking of this natural part of herself that did not have the opportunity to participate in life and to grow. Elizabeth compared this false self to a suit of armor, then said that her back had again been hurting and her physical therapist had said that the particular muscles involved tightened when she felt as if she were falling apart emotionally. The lower back muscles provided a kind of armor to hold her together. Elizabeth said the backache was therefore a physiological counterpart to what I described as a false-self personality organization.

A STRANGE ANOMALY: INCORPORATING AN OBJECT MEANS BEING INCORPORATED BY IT

Guntrip (1969) compared the concept of a regressed ego to that of Winnicott's true self. He remarked that the infant, faced with a toxic environment, withdraws to a passive state associated with the phantasy of a return to a womblike security. His view is based on Fairbairn's description of the internal object world. Fairbairn (1941) pointed out that the internalization of an object resulted in a strange anomaly: one incorporated and identified with an internal object while feeling incorporated by that object. In other words, when one internalizes an object, one feels incorporated by it. This process is associated with identification with the object, in which one feels incorporated by it. It will be recalled that Elizabeth felt an urgent need to evacuate inner contents whenever she felt claustrophobic. The symptom fits Fairbairn's idea. She felt trapped inside an object—whether it is a relationship, a meeting, or a train—which made her feel that the object was trapped within her. The object she felt trapped within symbolized the internal object. Similarly, the contents trapped within her symbolized an internal object.

Guntrip drew on Fairbairn's notion that the internalization of an object is accompanied by a phantasy of being incorporated or returning to an intrauterine state to advance his own view that the libidinal self related to internal objects undergoes a further split into an active, demanding oral self and a passive, regressed self state returning to a womblike security.

REACHING THE REGRESSED EGO

As Elizabeth's therapy focused on the area of a false self shielding the true self, she became more aware of her states of withdrawal. She said that as a child, she had a large wooden crate. She painted and decorated it to resemble a small house. She brought the box to her room or the backyard or in the front of her home. She sat in it for hours, experiencing it as a sanctuary that provided security. She had her own room, but she never felt securely closed in. The box was just large enough for her to fit into, and being inside it made her feel protected from the outer world. She now felt that the secure state she experienced within the box was strange and not based on reality, in that it afforded no real protection from the outer world and was no more effective than her own room in providing privacy. I remarked that the significant withdrawal was not hiding inside a box but rather withdrawing a part of herself and that the box represented that part of her mind into which she withdrew. The inner act of withdrawal for security was played out through the hiding in the box, which in turn reinforced the inner state of withdrawal. Although people could reach her inside her box, they were not so successful at reaching her in the inner world. In the box play, she pretended to be out of reach, but this very pretense disguised the fact that the same play was absolutely real in relationship to her emotional life.

Elizabeth now thought about other situations in her life that represented her internal state of withdrawal. In the past, every weekend she would stay home, describing her state of mind as "vegging out." Mornings continued to be difficult for her. She would pull the covers over her head, dreading getting up. In a state of extreme anxiety months earlier, she had been unable to arise. I explored carefully whether her withdrawal was an expression of the depressive position and the conflict around hate, or an expression of an earlier schizoid position and basic ego weakness. A patent may perceive the world as persecutory, standing between the patient and whatever he desires. It is as if the bad object stole the good object from the patient's grasp. Fear or guilt over aggression may cause the patient to withdraw from the persecutory object world. This is a problem of the depressive position. Elizabeth showed no evidence of the extreme idealization or devaluation that accompanies problems around hatred. It was not the world that seemed terrible or forbidding; she had a realistic view of it. When she felt strong, she asserted herself appropriately and was highly successful. Thus there was much accumulated evidence that her problems were not centered on the depressive positions. It was not that the world seemed persecutory but that she felt weak and too vulnerable to manage the ordinary stress of living. I interpreted that the backache also reflected her wish to regress and withdraw, not to have to deal with the world.

THERAPEUTIC REGRESSION

Guntrip (1969) emphasized that ego weakness refers to a basic relentless sense of fear, lack of self-confidence, weakness, and shame over weakness. Such ego weakness may be found in seemingly able, high-functioning people. Guntrip described a surgeon who had a successful practice for twenty years, was well respected by colleagues, but had one of the most undermined personalities he had ever treated. The feeling of weakness arises for such patients, not from generalized poor ego functioning, as in the case of borderline patients, but from a lack of feeling for one's own identity or reality. It is the failure to be loved fully as an autonomous being and a deficiency in mirroring that result in the basic fear, lack of confidence, and shame associated with ego weakness. Patients like Elizabeth split off and repress their basic ego weakness. The antidependent defenses permit the central ego to function as an adult, but with severe anxiety. Elizabeth's central self was comprised of obsessive-compulsive neurotic defenses that allowed her to function on a high level. Relationships were threatening because they exerted a regressive pull of the withdrawn, regressed ego that longed for contact but feared impingement and rejection. The fact that the regressed ego remains split off from the remaining personality to preserve autonomy means there can be no progress toward growth or maturity. For Elizabeth, the object was not persecutory or abusive. Rather, it was a look that did not see her, that turned away from her needs and focused critically on her autonomy. As she reentered the world of human relationships, there was the awakening need for mirroring and the dread that she would not be seen or the object would turn away or reject her.

As Elizabeth's regressive needs emerged in the transference, she habitually came to sessions late or heightened her intellectualized or obsessive style of presentation. I repeatedly interpreted her fear of merger and of being seen. Her neediness emerged more directly as she arrived with numerous feelings, questions, or problems and feared there was not enough time to discuss them. At the end of the session, when I told her our time was over, she always tried getting in another last sentence. She became aware that she was reliving feelings about her mother tucking her in for bed. The mother had stopped in the emotionally troubled brother's room first and spent a lot of time discussing his problems and putting him to bed. She then went into Elizabeth's room, exhausted and impatient. Elizabeth had never protested or acted out her wish for her mother to stay longer. In our relationship, she now increasingly protested about the separation as she relived the feelings of rejection by her mother.

Throughout most of the treatment, Elizabeth sat in a chair where she could see my face. During this period of therapeutic regression, however, she sometimes chose to lie on the couch. She emphasized that it was not because her back ached nor because she wished to facilitate free associations but because she wanted to relax. She also did not want me to sit behind her in the classical analytic position, but rather to sit where she could continue to see my face. Thus the use of the couch served a developmental purpose for therapeutic regression, a vehicle for expressing a need for ego care, to rest, to be without doing, as opposed to the classical purpose of uncovering.

The cases of Edward (see Chapter 12) and Elizabeth provide contrasting examples of seemingly obsessive-compulsive neurotic patients. Though both had underlying schizoid core issues, for Edward there were also important depressive position themes. For Elizabeth, the schizoid factors were dominant. Edward required much interpretation along with holding, whereas Elizabeth required mostly holding and some interpretation. Edward struggled to retain a good object in the face of his aggression, whereas Elizabeth struggled with issues of the true and false self. Although Edward accommodated a great deal to his environment and there were false-self aspects to his character, he did not suffer from a false-self personality organization as did Elizabeth.

14

THE TREATMENT OF A SEVERELY ACTING-OUT PATIENT

Borderline states may be related to conflicts around the depressive position. The borderline patient who suffers from deprivation fears that his hate will destroy the object. According to Winnicott (1956), deprivation implied that the patient had something that was lost. Antisocial behavior often is an expression of deprivation. For Winnicott, stealing in childhood is often an act of protest. The infant who had lost a good object or a period of satisfactory nurturance feels the loss to be a theft. It therefore takes back what had been stolen and what it has a natural right to.

Winnicott related withdrawn behavior to privation. In this case, there is hardly a sense of loss because the patient never felt he had anything to lose. There is little protest, which means there is little hope. The patient has no idea what he misses. For Winnicott, privation and withdrawal are more serious than deprivation and acting out. Privation results in a deficit in the internal good object and is often related to the schizoid condition. Privation is thus felt as an empty core. This schizoid emptiness is more primary than depressive emptiness that is related to hating and expelling an internal object. In schizoid emptiness, the object has never been sufficiently internalized. If an infant experienced a complete loss of good object relations, it would likely fail to thrive or survive.

Fairbairn's (1940) theory of the schizoid position as the core of the ego underlying the depressive condition implies a continuum between privation and deprivation.

Jean-Paul Sartre (1943) described how the self originates and emerges in the gaze of the other. In an earlier publication I (Seinfeld 1991b) described how the self is affirmed by the mirroring of the other but also how it is objectified, becomes the object of the other, and is therefore captured in the reflection of the mirroring object. This objectification in turn propels the infant to escape being the object of the other and to begin to sort out who it is from whom it is seen to be. The sense of being an object of the other results in the consciousness of being seen.

R. D. Laing (1959) applied Sartre's existential phenomenology to understanding the psychodynamics of borderline and schizoid states. Laing referred to a threatened or endangered sense of self as ontological insecurity. The self is endangered by the threats of engulfment, impingement, and petrification. The latter threat is the dread of being transformed into the object of the other. Ontological insecurity is the basis of the secret self. The secret self becomes a regressed self when faced with the three basic threats described by Laing.

The following case history provides a clear example of onto-logical insecurity, privation, and deprivation. The patient, Pamela, originally developed a false self organization that was later defended by antisocial behavior. She is in her mid-twenties and has been in therapy for eight years. Pamela was seen once weekly for the first year, twice weekly for five years, and lately once weekly. She originally came to therapy for overall poor social functioning.

PERSONAL HISTORY

Pamela grew up in an intact family with an older brother. Her maternal grandparents and aunts lived in the same apartment building as her family. Pamela's mother described her as a cooperative, nearly angelic child. She enjoyed dressing and grooming her daughter and showing her off to neighbors and friends. Everyone marveled at how pretty, perfect, and cooperative Pamela was.

Pamela was an astute child and was keenly aware of everything that went on around her, yet she was seemingly unperturbed by the familial chaos. Her father, an alcoholic, would become fanatical about religion when he intermittently quit drinking. Her parents fought constantly. Pamela screened out the fights and felt detached from the familial situation. She felt that she observed the family life through a television screen and that she was untouched by the craziness. She resembled Martin James's (1986) child who undergoes premature ego development resulting from impingement in the first months of life. James stresses that such infants become hypervigilant. He described a child who won an award as a baby for seeming so alert and precocious but, in fact, had suffered premature ego development from traumatic impingement. Pamela reported that she had been admired as an alert, perfect, precocious infant. James states, "Premature ego development would imply that the infant, during the phase of primary narcissism, took over the functions from the mother in actuality or started as though to do so. This would not be phase adequate under the age of three months" (p. 107).

The caregiver provides a protective shield from inner and outer impingement. If the parent fails in this function, the baby creates its own protective shield, often described by patients as a screen through which they perceive the impinging world. This may well describe how the regressed ego originally splits itself off from the exciting oral dependent libidinal ego.

Pamela was placed in nursery school and exhibited behavioral problems there. She refused to obey the teachers and had tantrums if they attempted to correct her. Her mother was surprised to learn of these problems and eventually removed Pamela from the school. During her childhood, Pamela was discouraged from making friends, attending after-school activities, or going to camp. If she fought or didn't get along with another child, her mother believed it was Pamela's fault and insisted that she attempt to befriend the other child. If Pamela became good friends with someone, her mother found something wrong with the other child and ridiculed the friendship. Her mother never expected her to do chores, clean up her room, or make her bed, nor did she praise Pamela if she did these things. However, when she was angry at Pamela, she would criticize her for her lack of responsibility.

Her father, a domineering man, deserted the family during Pamela's adolescence. While at home, he insisted that Pamela go to church every Sunday and read the Bible. Her father was especially strict during periods when he quit drinking. She was relieved when he would return to drinking because he would no longer care what she did.

Her parents found her to be a perfect child except for a period around the age of 2 or 3 when she refused to sleep alone in her room and cried until they brought her into their bed. This went on for some time, and Pamela never became a good sleeper. When she was made to sleep in her own bed, she would cry until her mother came and secretly turned on a television or radio. There were also rare instances when Pamela had a temper tantrum. Her parents, however, felt this was out of character and either immediately gave in to what she wanted or beat her.

In elementary school Pamela was timid and was picked on by her peers. At first, her parents restricted her from going out to play, but later, when they wanted her to go out, she resisted. She would spend most of her time in her room doing artwork, reading, or watching television. When she started junior high school, she remained reclusive and feared joining in after-school activities. She projected the aggression provoked by her family life onto the outer world and perceived it as threatening and dangerous.

Her parents felt that everything changed when Pamela was 14 and was caught shoplifting. Her mother was ashamed and didn't want to appear in public; her father told Pamela that she must be innately bad and should read the Bible every day to overcome her nature. Pamela felt that her father's designation of her as bad was accurate yet felt a certain inner pleasure in her mother's shame. She thought of how her mother had shown her off as a little angelic doll, but now she had become a devil child. At the same time, she had felt guilty about hurting her mother and had comforted her by saying how terrible she felt. Her mother cried, reminding Pamela of how she gave her whatever she asked for. Following this, however, her mother spoke to Pamela's father about reducing the punishment. Pamela had felt guilty about hurting her mother but felt pleasure and a sense of power that she had so influenced her. Although she genuinely had felt guilty, she also had found herself using her guilt to get her own way. While professing her guilt to her mother, another part of her had looked on detachedly and thought, "It's working; she's feeling bad and is now making up—it's perfectly predictable." This detached, observing part of herself looked on coldly and calculatedly, yet she had felt guilty about this attitude. She had wondered, "Do I feel guilty over what I did, or is it all a game? Am I acting just to get my way? Maybe I am a devil's child."

Pamela continued to get into trouble. She made friends with the kids in school who cut classes and used alcohol and marijuana and joined them in their acting out. She thought of herself as a "bad" kid, and there was a certain honor among her peers in this designation.

When Pamela was 16, her father left and moved in with another woman. Her mother had blamed Pamela for the breakup, saying that her father could no longer tolerate her behavior. Pamela knew there were marital problems of long duration but nevertheless felt that her problems had contributed to her father's departure. At the same time, she had felt pleased that he left because she would enjoy more freedom. Her mother had her own separation difficulties. Although she was angry at Pamela, she needed her. Her mother overindulged her, buying whatever Pamela wanted, allowing her to cut school, setting no limits.

In her twenties Pamela found boyfriends who would play the caretaking role that her mother performed. She would live with a boyfriend when she did not get along with her mother. When she and the boyfriend quarreled, she would return to her mother. It was at this point that Pamela sought therapy. Pamela had stopped attending high school at the age of 15 and quit altogether at the age of 16. She could not maintain a full-time job. She fought constantly with her mother, had been caught stealing, and occasionally used alcohol and marijuana.

BORDERLINE AND SCHIZOID FEATURES OF THE PERSONALITY

Pamela was an unusual patient in that she manifested both borderline and schizoid characteristics. An important distinction between these diagnoses is that the borderline patient suffers from generalized ego weakness (Kernberg 1975), whereas the schizoid usually does not. However, the schizoid patient experiences a split in the ego, whereby one part of the personality may stand over and above the other part and describe it with astute insight, in the manner of an observing ego, but have little influence over it. This observing ego is detached from the remaining personality and from genuine emotion, does not feel real, and is described as a false self. For instance, some anorexic patients can discuss their eating disorders with insight and clarity, yet may be presenting themselves to the interviewer in a disarming manner that protects the underlying disorder.

Pamela suffered from generalized ego weakness, as manifested in her inability to attend school, her poor impulse control, her judgment lapses, her abuse of drugs and alcohol, and her excessive dependence on others. At the same time, a schizoid split could be seen in the detached self that coldly observed her guilt reactions. Pamela was subject to intense, histrionic feelings, while another part of her remained detached. Her false self also was apparent in the charming but detached manner she used to relate to me. She exhibited borderline rage, but not with the frequency typical of the borderline patient.

Borderline patients like Pamela sometimes have underlying schizoid pathology, but it is unusual to find both borderline and schizoid factors dominating the surface of the personality. Given the extent and severity of Pamela's severely impaired ego functioning, I originally addressed interventions to the primitive defensive structure (Kernberg 1975). At the same time, I provided a holding relationship to allow for the emergence of the true self and underlying schizoid vulnerability. The ego had to be strengthened with enhanced separation-individuation to allow for the expression of the basic schizoid dilemma. In this first phase of treatment, holding served interpretation. The therapist's interventions are tolerated here because the patient experiences the support of an empathic object relationship. If the therapist interprets without providing supplemental support, the patient feels attacked and confronted. Later in the treatment, as the schizoid vulnerability emerges, holding becomes the major therapeutic response. Interpretations are then directed toward the patient's resistances to a holding object relationship.

PAMELA'S AVOIDANT, WITHDRAWN BEHAVIOR

In our first sessions, Pamela said she came to therapy because her life was not going anywhere. She admitted that she barely functioned. I asked how she felt about this, and she enthusiastically described her efforts at job hunting. It was my sense that the enthusiasm foreclosed the possibility of serious discussion of this issue as a problem. During the first months of treatment she was inconsistent about keeping appointments. She came for a few sessions, then missed without calling to cancel. She called days later with an excuse, saying she now wished to come. When she was in the midst of a conflict with a boyfriend, peers, or her mother, she avoided sessions. She did not respond to problems with reflection but rather by acting out. Thus, if her boyfriend stood her up, she was likely to find another man to sleep with. She might then let her boyfriend know, and they would argue or even come to blows. If her mother angered her, she went out drinking and placed herself in dangerous situations. She did not reflect on these problems when she was in the midst of acting out, but she did call in an emergency when the acting out led to trouble and she needed to respond. She did not want to understand why she was in trouble, yet was rather desperate to figure out how to act her way out of it. During such phone calls I rarely told her what to do—unless she was in immediate or extreme danger—but encouraged her to think about which of her options was the least dangerous to act on. This approach was tolerable for her because the end result would still be action; however, she at least began to reflect upon the various potential actions. The holding function here was both availability for the phone calls and permission to play with the possibilities for actions.

ACTING OUT AS A DEFENSE AGAINST SCHIZOID WITHDRAWAL

Pamela's acting out presented a therapeutic dilemma. In the case of a primarily borderline patient, the therapist might hold to the therapeutic frame in terms of scheduling, communicating only during sessions and interpreting the patient's behavior as a defense against abandonment anxiety (Masterson 1976). The therapist would thereby follow Freud's recommendation of insisting that the patient put all feelings into words, not actions. This is the essence of the therapist's paternal function.

In Pamela's case, her acting out was so pervasive that I understood it to reflect an underlying state of schizoid withdrawal. Fairbairn (1941) said when a patient's outer object relations are unsatisfactory, there is a withdrawal to internal object relationships. Pamela's clinging and demanding behavior toward objects could be understood in contrasting ways. From Fairbairn's view of the schizoid dilemma, she was desperately struggling to remain connected to objects and to counteract the tendency to withdraw. From an American object relations understanding of borderline phenomena, her clinging was a defense against separation. The intervention most suitable for the schizoid problem would be that of holding, and the intervention appropriate for the borderline problem that of interpretation. The severity of Pamela's urgent histrionic clinging pointed to a desperate struggle to remain in contact. She ran from her disappointing mother to her disappointing friends, from her disappointing friends to her disappointing boyfriends, from her disappointing boyfriends to her disappointing mother, from her disappointing mother to me. For Pamela, being alone threatened objectlessness. I believed that she desperately endeavored to stay in contact to fight off her own regressive longing to withdraw from object relations (Guntrip 1969). It was my sense that insisting on the classical frame and interpreting would have left her in an objectless state. I therefore provided a holding environment of availability. When she telephoned after not showing up or canceling, I spoke to her or rescheduled. If she called in an emergency, I provided an emergency appointment. There were occasions when I saw her beyond the scheduled 45 minutes, sometimes for 90 minutes, once for 2 hours.

SUPPORTING THE NEED FOR AN OBJECT

Pamela sometimes described in fragmented fashion the various relationships she clung to or fled from. If I were interviewing from the standpoint of the paternal function, I might have remarked upon her avoidance of focusing on one specific disappointment. Instead I said, "It is my sense that being left alone is utterly terrifying. You feel the way an infant might if left alone for too long. This is an issue most basic—survival—no one is there to help. Instead of giving up, you actively do something. Disappointed in someone, you demand what you feel you need or you seek someone else to hold on to. You fight for survival."

In this initial intervention, I did not interpret defenses against abandonment depression but instead focused on the threat of annihilation and supported the need for an object, any object at all, for survival. The intention was both revelatory (of annihilation and survival) and supportive of connecting. It was only after this basic anxiety became manageable that I could address the defenses against abandonment and separation.

THE INTERPRETATION OF PROJECTION

The interventions described provided the holding relationship that served as a foundation and support for the interpretations addressing her ego weakness and primitive defenses. During the first year of treatment, Pamela did not describe her acting out as a problem. She projected split-off and unconscious conflicts onto other persons. Kernberg (1975) distinguished projection from projective identification. In projection, the patient projects unwanted feelings, thoughts, or impulses onto the other and attempts to distance himself from the other to be rid of him. In projective identification, the patient feels a sense of oneness with the person he projected the feelings onto and typically pressures the other to have the same feelings.

> *Pamela*: The other day I passed some local kids. I know some of them, but not well. I thought of going over to talk but thought they were thinking of me as a real pothead and dropout. They all looked snotty. I said to myself, "screw you," and walked on. That's why I only go to see friends I get high with.

Therapist: Did they actually say anything to you or look at you in a strange way? Could you describe it?

Pamela: (laughs) Well, their eyes didn't pop out of their heads. They didn't say anything. Actually, the one I knew said hello.

Therapist: Then it sounds like you're describing your thoughts about their thoughts. You imagine that they think you're a pothead or dropout. They might but they might not. There's no evidence either way. It's you who think that.

Pamela: Most of the time I don't care what anyone thinks. But occasionally it bothers me and I do think that way. Those times alone at night thinking, "Where is my life going?"

INTERPRETING PROJECTION IN THE TRANSFERENCE

In the above example, the patient hardly knew the persons described as feeling negatively about her, so it was clear to the therapist that the patient was projecting her own negative thoughts about herself onto them. If she knew them well and believed they thought negatively of her, it would be more difficult for the therapist to know whether she was correct or whether she had utilized projective identification. Betty Joseph (1987) believed that projection and projective identification are most effectively interpreted in the transference–countertransference situation. The therapist can be more aware of the interaction and his own feelings and responses.

Pamela: I screwed up. You're not going to like it. I didn't go to work; I overslept. My boyfriend and I went downtown. It was a wonderful day. We had a picnic in the park, and John bought me some new clothes. I drank too much. The next day I woke up late again. I figured it's better to call in sick than go in late. They can't say anything if I'm sick, can they? Are you angry? You're not saying anything.

Therapist: You think of the bosses getting angry and me being angry. What makes you think that?

Pamela: It would be only natural. You try to help and I keep screwing up.

Therapist: When you thought of me as angry, what did you feel about me and this relationship?

Pamela: Afraid to come. I almost missed today.

Therapist: I noticed you were a little late. Was there a connection?

Pamela: The taxi came late. But yes, I dallied and left just enough time to get here.

Therapist: Thinking I was angry made you dally and thinking the boss was angry made you miss work. You act in such a way that you believe makes the other angry, and then you stay away and distance yourself.

Pamela: It sounds almost intentional.

Therapist: I'm not implying that. Sometimes you may not be thinking about something, but it may be expressed through your actions. Remember the old saying "Actions speak louder than words"? We might rephrase it as "Actions speak in place of words."

INTERPRETING ABANDONMENT ANXIETY

Early in treatment, the patient might project onto the therapist a negative superego reaction.

Pamela: There's something I'm thinking of telling you.

Therapist: What's keeping you from telling?

Pamela: You won't like it.

Therapist: Why do you say so? Have I given you a reason to think that?

Pamela: No. I guess I don't like it, so I think you won't. I got high last night.

We discussed how she had felt before getting high. Her boyfriend had left her alone to take care of his alcoholic sister, and she was angry that he put his sister first. She complained that he was not a man, always being at the beck and call of his family. She wanted to know if he was right to behave that way and what his problems were.

The key phrase in all she said was that her boyfriend "left her alone." Pamela did not have the capacity to be alone and would have been enraged no matter what the boyfriend's reason. The fact that his behavior was realistically problematic gave her justification to express and act out her rage. The attempt to convince the therapist to join her in blaming the boyfriend only served to support her efforts to avoid being alone. Actually, Pamela was improving at this point. In the past she could not have tolerated remaining home and would have gone outside, fought, pleaded, even cut her wrists (not in an effort to kill herself but in an attempt to cause self-mutilation). Now she got high and called numerous friends, complaining of her boyfriend's maltreatment. It was this small progress that indicated that she was ready for interpretations concerning abandonment depression.

> *Therapist*: There is likely some reality in your accusation that your boyfriend is putting his family first and neglecting you. This is the issue of whether he is mature enough for an intimate relationship. It may be that the intensity of your feelings is not only about this reality situation but also about being left alone. If you could tolerate being alone, you might leave him and find a new boyfriend, or deal with him differently.
>
> *Pamela*: I feel terrible. I think of cutting my wrists, throwing myself from a window. Nothing seems good. I call my mother but she's no help. She's going out with her boyfriend tonight. She never has time.
>
> *Therapist*: When you're alone, it seems you feel like a child left by a mother. You may feel like hurting yourself because you feel she's away and because you're worthless or unlovable. There is a rejecting image of her. Your boyfriend and your mother of today both symbolize the mother you longed for as an infant. You are reliving now the feeling you had earlier described when you had been left alone as a child.
>
> *Pamela*: It is that way. It feels childlike. It takes over entirely. I can't concentrate or read or watch a movie. I'm terrified, then enraged. I don't care about my boyfriend or myself. He's far from perfect, but he does show he cares.
>
> *Therapist*: Yes. He takes care of his sister and neglects you, not because you're worthless but because of his own background and issues. Even if he didn't care—I'm not saying that's the case—it wouldn't be about you but his difficulties in caring.

This interpretation was wordy but important in helping her to distinguish internal from external objects. The patient must first have some understanding of the internal relationship before she can deal effectively with the external object. Pamela began to recall memories of being left alone, with no sense of when her mother would return. When Pamela was jealous that her boyfriend went to his family, she was reliving the feelings of abandonment when her mother visited her own parents or siblings and left Pamela alone.

SUPPORTING AUTONOMY STRIVINGS IN THE CONTEXT OF A WEAK EGO

The literature concerning borderline pathology (Kernberg 1975, Masterson 1976) emphasizes that clinging is a defense against separation and abandonment depression. The above intervention illustrated the importance of this viewpoint. However, clinging may also serve the client's beginning efforts at autonomy. As internal separation of self and object representations occur, there may be clinging to the external object to alleviate the separation anxiety. Such clinging is reflective of a rapprochement (Mahler et al. 1975). A person suffering from severe pathology initially expresses autonomous strivings within the context of a weak and dependent ego structure. The therapist therefore may have to support dependence that serves autonomy. Holding is provided for adaptive dependence and interpretation for maladaptive dependence.

Pamela depended on her mother or boyfriends to drive her to appointments. If they were unavailable, she took a taxi, sometimes for a few city blocks. I interpreted how walking or traveling independently meant going on her own steam and therefore was an act of separation. My office was only a few blocks from where she lived. If she could not get someone to drive her and the taxi arrived late, she was enraged. She once had to walk when the taxi did not come and spent the first part of the session cursing her mother, boyfriend, and the cabdriver for not caring. I interpreted that she felt abandoned when she had to come on her own. When she started to look for a job, she had her boyfriend drive her to the interviews. I did not interpret, because she needed this support to begin to act autonomously. In fact, given her severe phobic tendencies, she would not have gone

out without support. Therefore, I provided her with an interpretation of separation anxiety but did not repeat it continually.

   After Pamela went on a job interview, she ridiculed herself for
being so immature as to need her boyfriend to drive her. She wondered that if she couldn't go to an interview on her own, what was
the point. I noted that simply going on the interview was a sign of
increased autonomy and that it was understandable that she needed
support. The experience was new and she couldn't change everything at once. She replied that this interview was different from
previous experiences. She had been on interviews before but had not
been nervous, probably because she knew there was no chance of
getting the job. She thought her anxiety in this interview implied
that she was becoming more serious about working. It turned out
that she did not go to work at this time. She felt she was a failure,
saying she might as well give up. I did not address my intervention
around taking or not taking the job itself, but rather explored the
underlying issue of autonomy. I remarked that the fact that she experienced more anxiety was an indication that there was more of a
wish for autonomy. I said, "A parent may actually discourage a child
by pressuring her to become independent all at once, and that is what
you are doing to yourself." She replied that that was what her
mother had done to her. Winnicott (1972) said that the therapist's
holding may provide the patient with a revelation about childhood.
Pamela recognized that her mother's pressure to do everything at
once may have been her mother's way of unconsciously discouraging her because she was afraid Pamela would become independent
and no longer need her. Pamela had identified with this aspect of her
mother and now became her own "internal saboteur."

INTERPRETING PROJECTIVE IDENTIFICATION IN
THE TRANSFERENCE

Pamela sometimes expressed despair in the transference–countertransference situation. She said she had had a terrible fight with her
boyfriend, that they had come to blows. She had gotten drunk and
hadn't gone to look for a job the next day. She talked of how her
mother and boyfriend did not help. She said that there was little to

live for, that she might as well be dead. No one cared. She said that I cared, but as a professional; it was my job. She said that she felt hopeless, that her life would never improve. Then she asked if I was angry.

> *Therapist*: What makes you ask? Have I given you that impression?
> *Pamela,*: I don't think so. I just think you would be angry or disappointed that I'm still stuck after so many years.
> *Therapist*: You may feel that way, so you imagine I do.
> *Pamela*: That's true. I feel I'm not getting anywhere.
> *Therapist*: You said no one is helping. You probably feel that way here as well.
> *Pamela*: I guess we're both stuck.
> *Therapist*: It could be that you're consciously trying to create a sense of despair in both of us. I'm not saying this is intentional, or that the feelings aren't genuine. It's my sense that sometimes you feel hopeless about both of us—that we're worthless as a therapeutic team.
> *Pamela*: It's something that comes over me. Not only with you, but with my boyfriend and mother. Anyone I'm close to.
> *Therapist*: It may be that even though it feels bad, there's something safe about it. Being stuck also means being stuck together, being stuck with the problems about your family, not going anywhere, not separating.

Pamela was actually beginning to take minuscule steps at separation. She had found a part-time job, had moved into an apartment with her boyfriend, began doing her own shopping and laundry. She therefore felt threatened with abandonment by the internal parental object. She created despair in the transference-countertransference situation to assure me that she would not change, that we were stuck, so that I would not abandon her.

REPEATING INSTEAD OF REMEMBERING IN THE TRANSFERENCE–COUNTERTRANSFERENCE

The treatment of the severely disturbed patient is fraught with frustration and helplessness. After finding a job and working longer than the usual few weeks, Pamela repeatedly complained of her persecutory female boss. I pointed out that up to a point, a boss was by definition a persecutor, in the sense of checking that the workers came and left on time, did their work, didn't overuse the phone for personal calls, and so forth. I said that some bosses simply do their job, but others may derive a sense of sadistic satisfaction above and beyond what the job requires. Pamela thought that her boss fit this description. I pointed out that her mother might also have been overly controlling, so that the boss might stand for her mother.

Pamela sometimes came in and told me of incidents in which she was quite provocative toward the boss. She would then complain, "Louise [the boss] thinks she's the queen. Everyone treats her that way. She takes as long for lunch as she pleases. She talks on the phone. She leaves early. Everyone worships her and the big boss, Mr. Cotter, doesn't say a word. But if I do anything like that, she immediately is on my back or she tells him."

She behaved similarly in the transference situation. She came in late, canceled without calling. At times, I found myself identified with her supervisor and similarly thinking of her as a malingerer. Once I became so carried away by countertransference that I said her boss would be justified in firing her for her acting out. As a child, when Pamela was late or disobedient, her mother had directed her father to punish her. Pamela said, "My father would kill me." She induced this situation in the workplace as the female supervisor told the male owner of the company about her acting out and in the transference situation as I found myself empathizing with her supervisor and lecturing her.

Pamela was beginning to separate and individuate. She provoked her internal objects to persecute her in order to reassure herself that they still cared and did not abandon her. Fairbairn (1958) described a patient whose parents attacked her if she expressed any of her own feelings or opinions. He went on, "It is, accordingly, interesting to note that, as the transference situation developed, [the patient] began to beg me to kill her." Fairbairn's patient said, "You would kill me if you had any regard for me," adding, "If you don't kill me, it means you don't care" (p. 79).

Thus Pamela repeated the early childhood situation by telling me how badly she treated her boss-mother and inducing me to punish her as her father had. On some level, she felt that if I lectured or attacked her, then I, as the father, still cared about her and was not abandoning her.

THE FEAR OF SUCCEEDING IN HER OWN NAME

Pamela and her boyfriend were evicted from their apartment for not paying their rent, and she had to return to her mother. She also was fired from her part-time job after a year, the longest she had ever worked at one place. She had been in treatment for six years and I felt doubtful that she could improve. Nevertheless, there were small indications of progress.

One of Pamela's friends attended college but was not doing well. Pamela, who had dropped out of high school but had earned an equivalency diploma, wrote an English paper for this friend. Her friend received an A for the work and the professor had commented, "Bravo! Some improvement. The quality is quite a surprise!"

Pamela was proud. Maybe she was smart enough to go to college.

> *Therapist*: Maybe you were testing this out, doing a paper in the name of your friend. A safe way to see if you could do it.
>
> *Pamela*: (laughs) Yes. Then if I fail, she gets the blame.
>
> *Therapist*: Yes, and if you succeed, she gets the credit.
>
> *Pamela*: True. It is kind of stupid. I do all the work and she gets the praise.
>
> *Therapist:* My remark was not meant to criticize.
>
> *Pamela*: I know. I'm criticizing.
>
> *Therapist*: But maybe that was the point. You may be as afraid of getting the credit as the blame. Doing it in her name, you not only fail to get the credit, you ridicule yourself for being stupid. Then, instead of thinking you're smart for getting an A, you think you're stupid for getting your friend an A.
>
> *Pamela*: I wonder why I need to think I'm stupid.
>
> *Therapist*: Why do you think? I have some thoughts about it, but first tell me your thoughts since they're most crucial.

Pamela: Maybe I'm afraid to do well in my own name. It's what you always say. I feel safe telling myself I'm stupid or a failure.

Therapist: I think it's that you fear being abandoned if you do well.

Pamela described how she had not been encouraged or supported for doing well in her childhood. If she did something badly, she never heard the end of it. She was not encouraged to study or do homework and if she asked for help, she was told to do it on her own, that she should not be a baby and try to get her parents to do it for her. They were uninvolved. But if she brought home a bad report card, her mother showed it to her father and he punished her.

Therapist: Then you were at least given attention. Now you do well, but in the guise of someone else, so you can call yourself stupid and not feel alone.

Pamela: My parents always called me stupid.

Therapist: By calling yourself stupid, you keep them with you.

Pamela: I guess it's good I did the paper, even if for someone else.

Therapist: Yes, you showed yourself you could do it in a way that felt safe.

INTERPRETING ABANDONMENT DEPRESSION IN THE TRANSFERENCE

Pamela avoided direct discussion of the transference. One of her appointments was for early Friday evening, and she regularly drank alcohol heavily afterwards. Putting on her coat to leave, she once said, "I'm going to get really bombed tonight."

I brought this up in our next session and explored what she was experiencing toward the end of the hour.

Pamela: I was thinking of everything I was going to do later that night. Getting high was only part of it. I was worrying where I would find my friends, what we would do. I was thinking of whom I'd call. I was in two places at once. I was here talking to you about my problems, while another part of me was planning the evening. I do that often. I'm never fully involved. When I'm with my friends, I'm also somewhere else.

Therapist: This being in two places at once could indicate anxiety about the situation you're in.

Pamela: I see that.

Therapist: Was there something we were discussing that disturbed you last time?

Pamela: I don't think it was the subject. It's relating itself. When you talk, I drift off. It's not only with you. It happened last week toward the end of the hour. I always drift off at the end.

Therapist: Are you reacting to having to leave?

Pamela: If I think about it, I hate it when you say the time is up. I used to get into serious things toward the end. You once said that I brought up the most important issues last because I feared discussing them. I don't believe you were correct. I simply brought up the most important issues last because I didn't want to go. You said we had to stop anyway. Then I just drifted off toward the end.

Therapist: So then you left before I said to leave. It may be that you evacuated me from your mind to protect yourself from feeling abandoned when I said it was time to stop.

Pamela: That's right. I was already outside in my mind by the time you said I had to leave.

Therapist: It may be that after you evacuated me from your mind, you felt empty inside. You then had to fill this by your heavy drinking, an urgent need to make plans and avoid being alone.

PAMELA'S IDENTIFICATION WITH HER FATHER AS AN EFFORT TO SEPARATE

Pamela began to write poetry and stories, which she then brought to me. She was ambivalent about this. She felt special that I valued her work enough to read it, but she also believed she should be able to make herself feel special and not depend on others. Her parents had not given her support and had discouraged her from getting it from outside sources. Thus she internalized their rejection of her need to be mirrored for her achievements and self-expression. I reminded her that the purpose of therapy was not to keep her dependent but to enable her to eventually be more on her own.

There was further indication that Pamela was becoming more autonomous. She applied to college full time for the fall semester. At the same time, she brought a tape of heavy metal music to a session so that I could understand what she enjoyed. After doing this, I asked her to tell me more about what she wanted me to understand. She replied that she was attracted to heavy metal guys. They were bad, rebellious, and tough. She thought of herself as a heavy metal girl. She said, "Do you ever notice that heavy metal guys don't take shit from anyone? They're also misogynist. Did you notice that in the lyrics?"

> *Pamela*: (laughing) Maybe they had smothering mothers and hate and reject all women. The essence of it is that if a girl asks for anything, they say, "Get lost, bitch."
>
> *Therapist*: What is it about them that you're drawn to?
>
> *Pamela*: I think I identify with them. My mother is a bitch. I am saying to her, "Get lost, bitch." But then again, to these guys I'm the bitch. Heavy metal guys hate controlling bitches, and I can be a controlling bitch. Especially when I'm afraid of being alone. My boyfriend puts up with it. I'm like my mother that way. I get it from her.
>
> *Therapist*: Where does the identification with the heavy metal guys come from?
>
> *Pamela*: My father. He had been a teenage gang member before he found respectability and religion. He was in a motorcycle gang. It was equivalent to being a heavy metal freak today. Once in a blue moon he told me of his old motorcycle adventures. If my mother was on his back, he ignored her or took her shit. But occasionally he'd become furious and tell her to get lost. At such times, I could see the Hell's Angel in him.
>
> *Therapist*: It sounds like your rebellious behavior was your way of being like your father. You could then tell your mother to get lost and go out into the world with your friends. By identifying with your father and becoming like the heavy metal guys, you're trying to break free from the inner dominating mother.

Pamela associated the paternal function with her father's rebellious history. Thus her rebellious behavior had an adaptive aspect. She was seeking out the paternal function to differentiate from the inner mother in the only way available. The father was himself not in the world. In fact, he was an alcoholic and could barely function. She found something in his history through which she could place him in the world. He was not autonomous, but she utilized his past experience with the motorcycle gang to symbolize separation or breaking away. The mother was actually in the world working much more than he. Thus, as Wright (1991c) points out, the father here is identified with the world, in the sense of being the world other than the mother, for purposes of differentiation and not because he is literally in the world more than the mother. However, the fact that the father was not a very autonomous person in his own right meant that she often had to identify with his negative traits, such as smoking, drinking, and delinquency.

AN EFFORT TO ADAPT WITHOUT FALSE-SELF CONFORMITY

Pamela raised the question of whether she could grow up emotionally to become a mature person but remain a rebel. Her mother had worried so much about everyone's opinion. If someone had insulted or mistreated Pamela as a child, her mother had automatically taken the other person's side and blamed Pamela. If Pamela had been justifiably angry at someone, her mother had told her to overlook it. Thus, as a child, Pamela had to be passive and obedient. When she rebelled in her adolescence, she no longer had felt like the passive, obedient child. She now wondered if she could be an autonomous person without being a conformist. She realized that the rebels she admired were not free because they could not take care of themselves and were slaves to drugs and alcohol.

Pamela was finally preparing to let go of the antisocial defense to face the schizoid false-self organization. Her parents had called her a thief long ago, and she had taken on this identity tag, becoming the baddest kid she could. This designation also fit with her phantasies of early childhood. She had felt robbed of her mother's love if she expressed autonomous strivings. Thus her acting out was her way of stealing back that lost love. When she was labeled a thief, she took on this identity because it fit with her phantasy. Sartre (1971) pointed out that the human tendency toward freedom can be manifested in our actively assuming the roles that others designate for us. Psychoanalytic theory, however, shows that the role assumed already has an unconscious basis. Pamela was also influenced toward antisocial behavior by the identification with her father discussed above. Her delinquency inevitably got her into trouble, which was experienced by her as a punishment for the destructive impulses against her mother. This antisocial depressive position functioning was a defense against her underlying false-self schizoid organization, which was now the focus of treatment.

SCHIZOID SPLITTING IN THE TRANSFERENCE

There was further evidence that Pamela was becoming more autonomous. She started college and, to my surprise, did not immediately drop out. She no longer panicked if her boyfriend left her alone. In fact, if he did, she went out with friends instead of sitting at home forlorn and depressed. This had the quality of a manic defense, but she clearly felt more autonomous and could, at least, use such a defense. The issue of closeness in the transference situation arose at this time. Pamela thought of coming to her session dressed in the "hot clothes" that she wore to clubs. She did not do so, deciding that it was not appropriate. She said she continued to feel insecure about her self-image. The insecurity centered on her appearance. Although she was pretty, she often felt that she was ugly. She was always thinking of heavy metal guys and had flirted with one the previous evening. She hardly knew him and had not found him especially interesting or attractive, but it was somehow extremely important that he had been interested in her. I asked what this was about.

> *Pamela*: Since it was the night before [this session], I think I was trying to distract myself from thinking of coming here. I was putting him between me and you—so I didn't have to think of what is happening.
> *Therapist*: What about what happens here that frightens you?
> *Pamela*: The positive feelings. You're the only person who helped me to become autonomous and to do what is right for myself.

The idea that you're helping me to grow up frightens me and makes me want to run away. But there is also the fear that you'll play with my mind and if I do feel close, you'll tell me to get lost. In reality I know I can trust you after all this time, but I feel insecure. I've been sexually obsessed with these heavy metal guys.

Therapist: Is that related to what you were saying about your feelings toward me?

Pamela: Lately, I feel close to you, especially since I've been discussing things like going to college. The closeness brings up sexual feelings. In my mind, I think of our relationship as ideal. You help me the way my parents should have. Sometimes, I wish I had a parent like you. I wish there were other people like you in my life. But then there are other feelings I have that make me anxious.

Therapist: Does that relate to what you said before—that I could tell you to get lost? Remember, you said the heavy metal guys tell the girl to get lost. You said that you think of them sexually to distract yourself from this relationship. On the other hand, you think of me as this ideal good parent—but then there are these other feelings— you associate me with the heavy metal guys who excite you but tell women to get lost.

Pamela: Mostly, I think of you as the ideal good parent. I know you're not like the heavy metal guys. But there are times when sexual feelings come up—I think of you that way.

Therapist: What is it that you mean by "that way"—could you elaborate?

Pamela: I mentioned it once—and it's not just about you. It's that when sexual feelings come up in this way. This is difficult to discuss. It's about violence, beating. Sometimes it's with the heavy metal guys, but sometimes the fantasy is with women. They beat someone. There is always domination. I think of you that way but then turn it off. There's also this fear of rejection. It's all mixed together. But when I have the excited feelings, I'm more fearful of rejection—that's why I turn the feelings off.

Therapist: The thing about rejection. I guess if you begin to feel sexual and dependent feelings toward me, you feel vulnerable. You tell me such feelings and I just sit and listen and ask how you feel. The very nature of this response may cause you to feel frustrated and rejected.

In the following sessions, Pamela became aware of schizoid splitting in the transference. She felt our relationship to be ideal when she drank. At first, she had erotic feelings, but these were submerged as she thought of all I did for her, that I was supportive and caring. She had felt this way about her grandfather. He was similar to a child himself and had indulged her. He met her every wish. Her mother always said he was wrapped around Pamela's finger. He was her candy man. He brought her candy, toys, gifts; he took her to the movies and to the park. She was close to him until she became an adolescent and began to develop sexually. He said she was no longer his little girl and withdrew. She felt this same way about me and her boyfriend. She believed that she drank to sustain this ideal feeling.

> *Therapist*: And what if you don't drink? Do feelings come up that disturb the ideal relationship?
> *Pamela*: The sexual feelings. I was thinking of something further. My mother always held me on her lap when I was little. It became uncomfortable. She pawed at me, kissing, pinching, touching me all over. I don't mean she abused me. But I thought of her as clawing me. Do you know how you say I fight with my mother for distance? Well, I believe this is why I needed the distance. The fighting started soon before my adolescence. Even before that, I went to my grandfather. I couldn't go to my father. He was either drunk or giving crazy religious sermons. He became punitive and rejecting if I did not do exactly what he believed.
> *Therapist*: It sounds as if keeping me in this ideal state is a way of staying in contact. If the disturbing, exciting, or rejecting feelings arise, it becomes more difficult for you to relate to me.

MIRRORING AND THE FEAR OF BEING SEEN

The development of the transference illustrated Fairbairn's theory of the underlying schizoid psychic structure. Fairbairn (1944) described how the idealized relationship to the external object served to split off the exciting and rejecting internal relationships. Pamela related to me as the ideal grandfather to defend against projecting onto me the exciting mother and the rejecting father. It was only after interpretations had helped her to become relatively autonomous and able to tolerate separateness that the split-off transferences could begin to emerge. Pamela first exhibited this readiness by expressing the need for mirroring, but in an eroticized fashion. In other words, I had interpreted her identification with her parents' rejection of her need to be mirrored when she brought her poetry and stories to our sessions. Shortly thereafter, she had wanted me to see her in her "hot clothes." There was a strong wish to be admired for beauty and a fear that I perceived her as ugly. Winnicott (1971c) noted that the urgent need to be mirrored as physically beautiful points toward failure in early mirroring, which is reflected in the sense that one is ugly. It was at this point that Pamela activated the early split-off bad object transferences, which must be worked through before the patient is able to express the early natural need for mirroring. I repeatedly interpreted the oscillation between the exciting and rejecting internal relationships as described above. The intervals between sessions became difficult for her as she relived the longing for the early object. Memories emerged of being left alone by her parents and withdrawing in a world of phantasy.

THE SUPPORTIVE RELATIONSHIP SERVING AUTONOMY

Pamela started college full time. Initially, she asked to reduce the frequency of our sessions because of her busier schedule and tuition payments. It is my experience that severely disturbed patients often want to cut back on their sessions when they take a major step in autonomous functioning. This is the patient's way of practicing separateness. I have found it wise to agree or the patient experiences the therapist as interfering with autonomy or not trusting that the patient can manage. Within a month, Pamela resumed our weekly sessions.

There was a question of how she would get to school. Pamela planned to drive but did not have her license yet and the school was not easily accessible to public transportation. She told me she would have to drive her mother's car or buy one and drive it without a license. I interpreted that her conflict about how she would get there was an expression of her fear of separating. I said that traveling was symbolic of separating. Doing it by driving without a

license was a way of acting out the phantasy that she was doing
something forbidden, against the law, by going to school. I said,
"You're acting out the phantasy that you are transgressing your
mother's law and that she is justified in punishing you." At times
she tried to argue, stating that she was a good driver and would not
have an accident. I replied, "I'm not saying this to try to control you
or to give you a lecture. It's my experience that when people begin
to do something that is right and important for themselves, but do
it the wrong way or attempt to take a shortcut, it often doesn't work
out." To my surprise, she said she knew what I meant, that it was
her experience as well.

In the above interventions, I fulfilled the paternal function in
terms of setting limits and interpreting her resistances to separating
from the mother. However, the paternal function had to be used in
conjunction with the maternal function. When I began to treat
Pamela, I was under the impression that she at first would have to
call a great deal but that later this would lessen significantly. This
was only partially true. Whenever she took a new developmental
step, she would have much greater need for telephone contact
because of a heightened fear of abandonment. There were occasions
when I was put off by her becoming more needy and returning to
dependence. This was particularly so if I had taken on more work
responsibilities in the interval since she had last gone through
dependence. Winnicott (1962) remarked that the therapist must
take into account his own scheduling and emotional availability
before allowing the patient to undergo an experience of regression.
Little (1990) said that Winnicott had a "waiting list" for his patients
already in treatment and that a patient had to wait his or her turn
until Winnicott could allow for the regression.

When the therapist takes on a severely disturbed patient for a
prolonged time, the therapist can decide when the first regressive
experience will occur. In the case of Pamela, the first dependent
experience was both the longest and most intense. However, with
each change in her life there was again a need for dependence, and
the timing was often less convenient for me. She sometimes picked
up in my tone that I was less than tolerant. She complained that I
was too busy, as her mother had been. I had paid attention to her
when she was very disturbed, but now that she was doing better, I

did not want to be bothered and expected her to be completely independent. She felt that I did not want her to be independent and therefore only rewarded her for dependence. At other times she felt that I wanted her to be completely independent because I was tired of treating her and wanted to be rid of her. I became aware that when she began to function more independently, she needed me even more to serve as a holding object. Once I did, she was reassured and soon no longer needed the extra contacts.

RELIVING THE CRITICAL GAZE OF THE BAD OBJECT

As Pamela began college, she became considerably more autonomous as she traveled to school and met new people. Her conflicts about mirroring came completely to the fore. She described feeling that other students looked at her critically, or talked among themselves about her. She had given a talk in a speech class and had received an A. The other students had looked enthused and had congratulated her. On the one hand, she was extremely excited and pleased, but on the other, she could not fully believe they thought so well of her. There were other occasions when students responded critically, competitively, or enviously. I noticed that she became especially anxious after receiving an A for an oral presentation. During one session she described meeting one of her mother's friends on the street and imagined that the woman was thinking negatively about her, in much the way she knew her mother to think badly of her. She experienced the woman's look as petrifying her into an object and realized that she was allowing her to make her feel this way. She imagined that her mother had told this woman everything that was wrong with her and the woman therefore saw her through her mother's eyes. I interpreted that Pamela was beginning to express her autonomous self for the first time. She was reliving the early need for her mother's mirroring and the ways that her mother had failed her. She was seeing that she could survive and also that she could sometimes be mirrored for the person she was. She was most frightened when she did well, because she feared the other would turn away, not see her. She could only be seen when she failed, but this meant being seen negatively. Later in this same session Pamela said that she felt close to me and that it frightened her. She said in all the years she had been seeing me, she had always felt detached, as if another self spoke to me. She felt this detachment with everyone. When she had told me of the adventures in her life, she had felt as if she were play acting. Sometimes she felt as if she felt upset in order to feel real and involved. Now, as she felt more connected, she was aware for the first time how detached she had always felt. For the first time, she felt really close to me, and it terrified her. It felt as if she were sinking into a bottomless pit of emptiness or need, and she felt like grabbing onto me so that she did not fall in and lose herself.

THERAPEUTIC REGRESSION

Pamela's feeling that she was falling into a bottomless pit indicated that she was experiencing regression in the transference. Guntrip (1969) pointed out that the regression can be destructive or thera-peutic, depending on whether the patient feels there is an object to regress to. Pamela's feeling of falling into a bottomless hole of emptiness refers to the fact that she begins to relive her early deprivation and emptiness in the transference. Falling signified letting go of her false-self organization that replaced the early caregiver and walled off her own needs.

In recent sessions, she stated that there have been occasions when she has felt close to me and then thought of stabbing me with a knife. They were not occasions when she was angry. Rather, she felt authentically close. Then the murderous thoughts would in-trude and she would think it was not good for her to be so close. This reminded her of occasions in her childhood when a calm and mature adult would be present and her mother would whisper to her how arrogant the person was and how she should be knocked off her high horse. Pamela felt that her thoughts about stabbing me were the expression of the inner mother that did not want her to have a good relationship.

Pamela is on the dean's list in college. She now takes public transportation to school. She broke up with her old boyfriend, feeling that he was too limited and had too many problems, but they remain friends. She now has a new boyfriend and is surprised that someone can treat her so well. At the same time, she mourns the relationship with her old boyfriend and realizes that, in mourning their relationship, she also mourns her mother. She remains free spirited.

References

Abraham, K. (1919). A particular form of neurotic resistance against the psycho-analytic method. In *Selected Papers*, pp. 303–311. New York: Brunner/Mazel, 1927.

_____ (1920). The narcissistic evaluation of excretory processes in dreams and neuroses. In *Selected Papers*, pp. 318–326. New York: Brunner/Mazel, 1927.

_____ (1921). Contributions to the theory of the anal character. In *Selected Papers*, pp. 370–392. New York: Brunner/Mazel, 1927.

_____ (1924). A short study on the development of the libido in the light of the mental disorders. In *Selected Papers*, pp. 418–502. New York: Brunner/Mazel, 1927.

Balint, M. (1968). Primary love. In *The Basic Fault: Therapeutic Aspects of Regression*, pp. 64–72. New York: Brunner/Mazel.

Benjamin, J. (1988). The first bond. In *The Bonds of Love*. New York: Pantheon.

Bion, W. (1962). *Learning from Experience*. London: Maresfield Library Reprints.

_____ (1967). *Attacks on Linking*. London: Maresfield Library.

Bollas, C. (1987). *The Shadow of the Object*. New York: Free Association.

Bowlby, J. (1958). The nature of the child's tie to his mother. In *Essential Papers on Object Relations*, ed. P. Buckley. New York: New York University Press, 1986.

Buber, M. (1958). *I and Thou*. New York: Scribner.

Bunting, M. (1992). *Guardian*. London: August 12.

Dupont, J. (1991). Introduction. In *The Clinical Diary of Sandor Ferenczi*, ed. J. Dupont, pp. xi–xxvii. Cambridge, MA: Harvard University Press.

Eigen, M. (1973). Abstinence and the schizoid ego. *International Journal of Psycho-Analysis* 54:495–498.

——— (1980). The significance of the face. In *The Electrified Tightrope*, pp. 49–60. Northvale, NJ: Jason Aronson, 1992.

Fairbairn, W. R. D. (1940). Schizoid factors in the personality. In *Psychoanalytic Studies of the Personality*, pp. 3–27. London: Routledge and Kegan Paul, 1952.

——— (1941). A revised psychopathology of the psychoses and psychoneuroses. In *Psychoanalytic Studies of the Personality*, pp. 28–58. London: Routledge and Kegan Paul, 1952.

——— (1943). The repression and the return of bad objects. In *Psychoanalytic Studies of the Personality*, pp. 59–81. London: Routledge and Kegan Paul, 1952.

——— (1944). Endopsychic structure considered in terms of object relationships. In *Psychoanalytic Studies of the Personality*, pp. 82–136. London: Routledge and Kegan Paul, 1952.

——— (1954). Observations on the nature of hysterical states. In *British Journal of Medical Psychology* 27:8–118.

——— (1958). On the nature and aims of psychoanalytic treatment. *International Journal of Psycho-Analysis* 39:374–385.

Ferenczi, S. (1920). The further development of an active therapy in psychoanalysis. In *Further Contributions to the Theory and Technique of Psycho-Analysis*, New York: Brunner/Mazel, 1926.

——— (1930). The principles of relaxation and neo-catharsis. In *Final Contributions to the Problems and Methods of Psycho-Analysis*, New York: Brunner/Mazel, 1955.

——— (1933). Confusion of tongues between adults and the child. In *Final Contributions to the Problems and Methods of Psycho-Analysis*, New York: Brunner/Mazel, 1955.

——— (1988). *The Clinical Dairy of Sandor Ferenczi*. Ed. J. Dupont. Cambridge, MA: Harvard University Press.

Freeman, L. (1972). *The Story of Anna O*. New York: Walker.

Freud, S. (1905). Fragment of an analysis of a case of hysteria. In *Collected Papers*, vol. 3, ed. A. Strachey and J. Strachey, pp. 13–133. New York: Basic Books, 1959.

——— (1914). Remembering, repeating and working through. In *Collected Papers*, vol. 2, ed. J. Riviere. New York: Basic Books, 1989.

——— (1915a). Observations on transference love. In *Collected Papers*, vol. 2, ed. J. Riviere. New York: Basic Books, 1959.

——— (1915b). Some character types met with in psychoanalytic work. In *Collected Papers*, vol. 4, ed. J. Riviere, pp. 318–344. New York: Basic Books, 1959.

_____ (1917). Mourning and melancholia. In *Collected Papers*, vol. 4, ed. J. Riviere. pp. 152–172. New York: Basic Books, 1959.

Freud, S., and Breuer, J. (1895). Fraulein Anna O. In *Three Studies on Hysteria*, ed. J. Strachey, A. Strachey, and A. Richards, pp. 73–102. New York: Penguin, 1974.

Greenberg J. R., and Mitchell, S. A. (1983). *Object Relations in Psychoanalytic Theory*. Cambridge, MA: Harvard University Press.

Grotstein, J. (1981). *Splitting and Projective Identification*. New York: Jason Aronson.

Guntrip, H. (1961). *Personality Structure and Human Interaction* London: Hogarth.

_____ (1969). *Schizoid Phenomena, Object Relations and the Self*. New York: International Universities Press.

_____ (1975). My experience of analysis with Fairbairn and Winnicott: how complete a result does psycho-analytic therapy achieve? In *Essential Papers on Object Relations*, ed. P. Buckley. New York: New York University Press, 1986.

Hinshelwood, R. (1989). *A Dictionary of Kleinian Thought*. Northvale, NJ: Jason Aronson.

Isaacs, S. (1948). On the nature and function of phantasy. *International Journal of Psycho-Analysis* 29:73–97.

Jacobson, E. (1964). *The Self and the Object World*. New York: International Universities Press.

James, M. (1986). Premature ego development: some observations on disturbances in the first three months of life. In *The British School of Psychoanalysis: The Independent Tradition*, ed. G. Kohon, pp. 101–116. London: Free Association.

Joseph, B. (1982). Addiction to near death. In *Psychic Equilibrium and Change*, ed. E. B. Spillius and M. Feldman, pp. 27–138. New York: Tavistock, 1989.

_____ (1985). Transference: the total situation. In *Psychic Equilibrium and Change*, ed. E. B. Spillius and M. Feldman, pp. 198–216. New York: Tavistock, 1989.

_____ (1986). Psychic change and the psychoanalytic process. In *Psychic Equilibrium and Change*, ed. E.B. Spillius and M. Feldman, pp. 192–202. New York: Tavistock, 1989.

_____ (1987). Projective identification—some clinical aspects. In *Psychic Equilibrium and Change*, ed. E. B. Spillius and M. Feldman, pp. 168–180. New York: Tavistock, 1989.

Josephs, L. (1992). *Character Structure and the Organization of the Self*. New York: Columbia University Press.

Kavaler-Adler, S. (1992). Mourning and erotic transference. *International Journal of Psycho-Analysis* 73:527–539.

Kelley, K. (1988). *The Home Planet: Images and Reflections of Earth from Space Explorers*. London: Macdonald Queen Anne Press.

Kernberg, O. (1975). *Borderline Conditions and Pathological Narcissism*. New York: Jason Aronson.

―――― (1980). *Internal World, External Reality*. New York: Jason Aronson.

Klein, M. (1935). A contribution to the psychogenesis of manic depressive states. In *Love, Guilt, Reparation and Other Works, 1921–1945*, pp. 262–289. New York: The Free Press.

―――― (1940). Mourning and its relation to manic depressive states. In *Love, Guilt and Reparation and Other Works, 1921–1945*, pp. 344–369. New York: Delta, 1975.

―――― (1946). Notes on some schizoid mechanisms. In *Envy and Gratitude and Other Works, 1946–1963*, pp. 1–24. New York: The Free Press.

―――― (1957). *Envy and gratitude*. In *Envy and Gratitude and Other Works, 1946–1963*, pp. 176–235. New York: The Free Press.

Kohut, H. (1971). *Analysis of the Self*. New York: International Universities Press.

Lacan, J. (1949). *Ecrits*. New York: W. W. Norton.

―――― (1955). The Freudian thing, or the meaning of the return to Freud in psychoanalysis. In *Ecrits*, pp. 114–143. New York: W. W. Norton, 1977.

Laing, R. D. (1959). *The Divided Self*. Middlesex, England: Penguin.

Little, M. (1986). On basic unity. In *The British School of Psychoanalysis: The Independent Tradition*, ed. G. Kohon, pp. 136–153. London: Free Association.

―――― (1990). *Psychotic Anxieties and Containment: A Personal Record of an Analysis with Winnicott*. Northvale, NJ: Jason Aronson.

Loewald, H. (1960). On the therapeutic action of psychoanalysis. In *The Work of Hans Loewald*, ed. G. Fogel, pp. 13–60. Northvale, NJ: Jason Aronson. 1991.

Masterson, J. (1976). *Psychotherapy of the Borderline Adult*. New York: Brunner/Mazel.

Mahler, M., Bergman, A., and Pine, F. (1975). *The Psychological Birth of the Human Infant*. New York: Basic Books.

Ogden, T. (1986). *The Matrix of the Mind: Object Relations and the Psychoanalytic Dialogue*. Northvale, NJ: Jason Aronson.

Rayner, E. (1991). *The Independent Mind in British Psychoanalysis*. Northvale, N.J.: Jason Aronson.

Rinsley, D. (1981). Object relations theory and psychotherapy with particular reference to the self-disordered patient. In *Technical Factors in the Treatment of the Severely Disturbed Patient*, ed. P. L. Giovacchini and L. B. Boyer, pp. 187–216. New York: Jason Aronson.

Rosenfeld, H. (1987). Destructive narcissism. In *Impasse and Interpretation*, ed. D. Tuckett, pp. 70–84. London: Tavistock

Sandler, J., and Sandler, A. M. (1978). On the development of object relations and affects. In *Essential Papers on Object Relations*, ed. P. Buckley, pp. 272–292. New York: New York University Press.

Sartre, J. P. (1940). *The Psychology of Imagination*. Secaucas, NJ: Citadel.

———— (1943). *Being and Nothingness*. New York: Washington Square Press.

———— (1960). *Critique of Dialectical Reason*. Vol. 1. London: Verso.

———— (1971). *The Family Idiot: Gustave Flaubert 1821-1857*. Vol. 1. Chicago: University of Chicago Press.

Scharff, J. S. (1992). The forgotten concept of introjective identification. In *Projective and Introjective Identification and the Use of the Therapist's Self*, pp. 49–83. Northvale, NJ: Jason Aronson.

Scharff, J. S., and Scharff, D. E. (1992). *Scharff Notes: A Primer of Object Relations Therapy*. Northvale, NJ: Jason Aronson.

Searles, H. (1965). Phases of patient–therapist interaction in the psychotherapy of chronic schizophrenia. In *Collected Papers on Schizophrenia and Related Subjects*, pp. 521–559. New York: International Universities Press.

Segal, H. (1981). Melanie Klein's technique. In *The Work of Hanna Segal*. Northvale, NJ: Jason Aronson.

Seinfeld, J. (1990a). The negative therapeutic reaction. In *The Bad Object: Handling the Negative Therapeutic Reaction*, pp. 3–20. Northvale, NJ: Jason Aronson.

———— (1990b). Intervention with the out of contact patient. In *The Bad Object: Handling the Negative Therapeutic Reaction*, pp. 163–188. Northvale, NJ: Jason Aronson.

———— (1990c). Manifestations of the bad internal object. In *The Bad Object: Handling the Negative Therapeutic Reaction*, pp. 21–60. Northvale, NJ: Jason Aronson.

———— (1991a). A framework for the empty core. In *The Empty Core*, pp. 3-26. Northvale, NJ: Jason Aronson.

———— (1991b). Captured in the reflection of the mirror. In *The Empty Core*, pp. 29-50. Northvale, NJ: Jason Aronson.

Shakespeare, W. (1988). *The Tragedy of Julius Caesar*. In *William Shakespeare: The Complete Works*, compact edition, ed. S. Well, G. Taylor, J. Jowett, and W. Montgomery. Oxford: Clarendon Press.

Stanton, S. (1991). *Sandor Ferenczi: Reconsidering Active Intervention*. Northvale, NJ: Jason Aronson.

Stewart, H. (1986). Problems of management in the analysis of a hallucinating hysteric. In *The British School of Psychoanalysis: The Independent Tradition*, London: Free Association.

Sutherland, J. (1963). Object relations theory and the conceptual model of psychoanalysis. *British Journal of Medical Psychology* 36:109–124.

———— (1989). *Fairbairn's Journey to the Interior*. London: Free Association.

Ticho, E. A. (1974). Donald W. Winnicott, Martin Buber and the theory of personal relationships. *Psychiatry* 37:240–253.

Volkan, V. (1987). *Six Steps in the Treatment of Borderline Personality Organization.* Northvale, NJ: Jason Aronson.

Winnicott, D. W. (1951). Transitional objects and transitional phenomena. In *Collected Papers: Through Paediatrics to Psychoanalysis*, pp. 229–242. London: Hogarth.

―――― (1954). Metapsychological and clinical aspects of regression within the psychoanalytic set-up. In *Through Paediatrics to Psycho-Analysis*, pp. 278–294. London: Hogarth.

―――― (1955). A case managed at home. In *Collected Papers: Through Paediatrics to Psycho-Analysis*, pp. 118–128. London: Hogarth.

―――― (1956). The anti-social tendency. In *Collected Papers: Through Paediatrics to Psycho-Analysis*, pp. 306–315. London: Hogarth.

―――― (1958). The capacity to be alone. In *The Maturational Processes and the Facilitating Environment*, pp. 29–36. New York: International Universities Press, 1965.

―――― (1960). Ego distortion in terms of true and false self. In *The Maturational Processes and the Facilitating Environment*, pp. 140–152. New York: International Universities Press.

―――― (1962). The aims of psychoanalytic treatment. In *The Maturational Processes and the Facilitating Environment*, pp. 166–170. New York: International Universities Press.

―――― (1963). The mentally ill in your caseload. In *The Maturational Processes and the Facilitating Environment*, pp. 217–229. New York: International Universities Press.

―――― (1971a) Creativity and its origins. In *Playing and Reality*, pp. 65–85. New York: Tavistock.

―――― (1971b) The use of object and relating through identification. In *Playing and Reality*, pp. 86–94. New York: Tavistock.

―――― (1971c) Mirror role of mother and family in child development. In *Playing and Reality*, pp. 111–118. New York: Tavistock.

―――― (1972). *Holding and Interpretation.* New York: Grove.

Wright, K. (1991a). The other's view. *In Vision and Separation: Between Mother and Baby*, pp. 23–38. Northvale, NJ: Jason Aronson

―――― (1991b). Symbol formation. In *Vision and Separation: Between Mother and Baby*, pp. 89–110. Northvale, NJ: Jason Aronson.

―――― (1991c). The role of the father. In *Vision and Separation: Between Mother and Baby*, pp. 111–126. Northvale, NJ: Jason Aronson.

―――― (1991d). Therapy and the self. In *Vision and Separation: Between Mother and Baby*, pp. 279–302. Northvale, NJ: Jason Aronson.

Index

Abraham, K., 55, 70, 135, 191
  depressive pathology and, 32
  on interpreting the loss of internal
    objects, 22–25
  on narcissistic personality disorders,
    21
  on object relations theory, 21
  on retaining interval object, 225
  on timing of interpretation, 25–27
Abused child, 66–67, 86–87, 199, 205,
  208, 212
Acting-out patient
  acting out as defense against
    schizoid withdrawal, 277–279
  adapting without false-self
    conformity, 291–292
  autonomy, 295–298
  borderline and schizoid features,
    275–276
  fear of success, 287–288
  identification with father, 289–291
  interpretation of projection,
    279–281
  interpreting abandonment anxiety
    and depression, 281–284,
    288–289

  mirroring, 294–295
  schizoid splitting in transference,
    292–294
  therapeutic regression, 298–299
  transference–countertransference,
    284–287
Addams, J., 177
Aggression, 36–38, 45, 63–64
Anal reactions, 22
Analytic space, 6
Analytic therapy, 55–57
Anger, 23
Anna O.
  and discovery of "talking cure,"
    177
  hysteria and, 178–188
  and social work, 177, 183
Anxiety, 35, 198–203
  separation, 59–60, 71–77, 230,
    281–284, 288–289

Balint, A., 8
Balint, M., 8, 42, 109, 112, 114, 131
  and Ferenczi, 93–94
  and libido, 57

307